¡UN DOCTOR POR FAVOR!

PAOLA MINA-OSORIO
MD, PHD

Why We Need
More Hispanic Physicians In The U.S.,
A Look At The Numbers And Beyond

First edition April 2020
ISBN: 978-1-7351728-0-4

Edited by Katharine Bernard
Cover illustration by Priyanka Shrivastava
Cover design by Joseph Polsin

The opinions expressed in this book are those of the author and do not
necessarily represent those of any of her past or present employers.

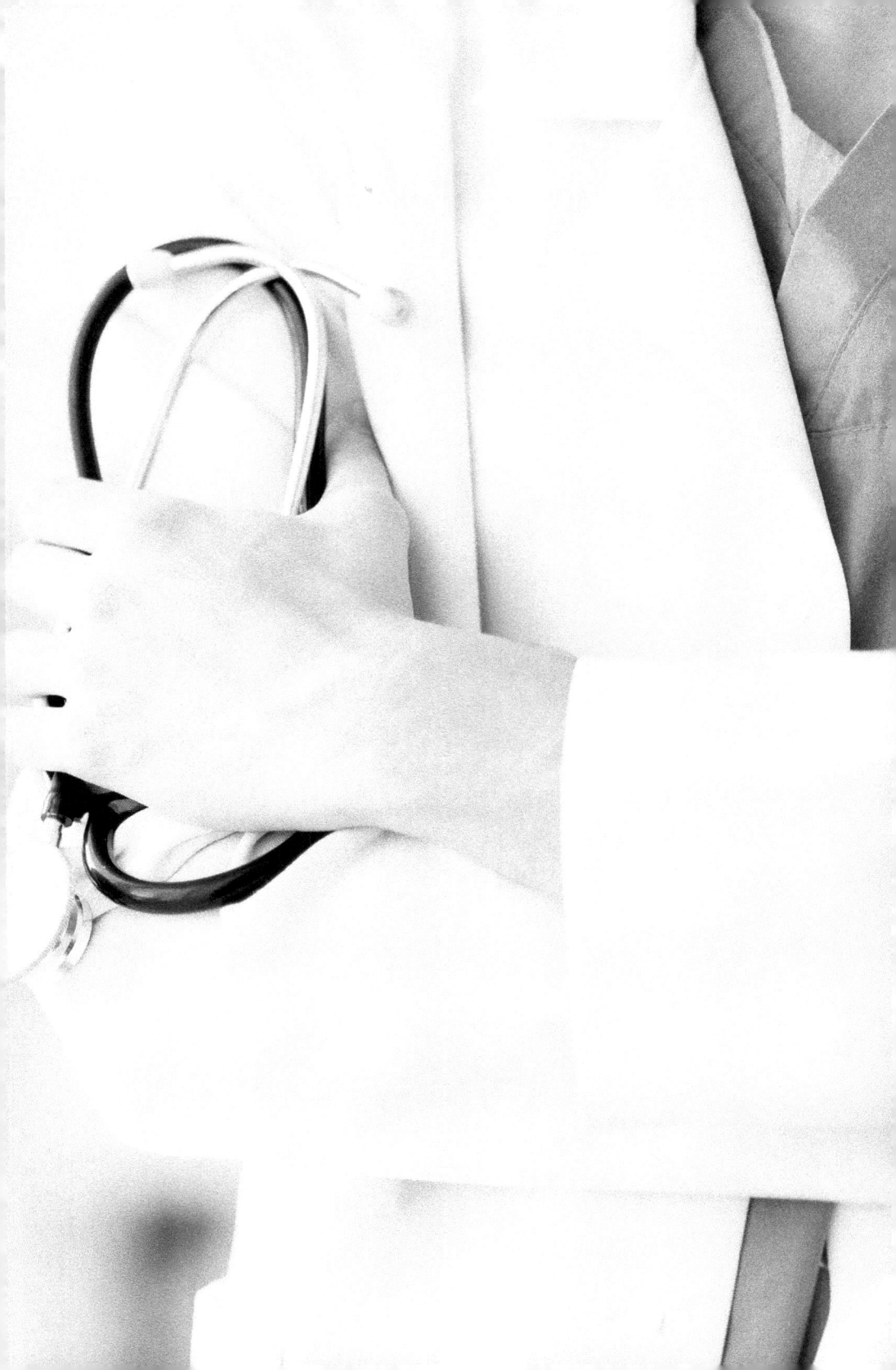

*To my father, who defeated poverty and inequality to become a doctor
who has saved many lives and shaped mine.*

*To my mother, who has been a model of strength and dedication,
as well as the most constant and supportive presence in my life.*

*To my husband, who is my rock, my companion and my biggest supporter.
He always reminds me that I can reach for the stars.*

*To my sister, who is always there for me.
She is educating the next generation of Ecuadorian physicians.*

*To all those who told me that becoming a doctor and a scientist
would be too hard, that it would take too long, or that it was impossible,
but mostly to those who said: Yes, you can!*

*To all Hispanics in the U.S., who dream of becoming doctors and will.
To those who look in the mirror and see themselves as part of the next
generation of Hispanic physicians in the U.S.*

TABLE OF CONTENTS

Chapter Two:

Hispanics Beyond the Numbers: Hispanic Racial Identity is Multidimensional

SECTION TWO: HISPANIC EDUCATIONAL ATTAINMENT

Chapter Three:

The Educational Pipeline by the Numbers: How early do the disparties begin?

SECTION THREE: WHY DO WE NEED MORE HISPANIC DOCTORS?

Chapter Five:

Hispanic Health by The Numbers

Chapter Six:

Hispanic Health Beyond The Numbers: Why do we need more Hispanic Doctors in the U.S.?

231 SECTION FOUR: STORIES OF HISPANIC PHYSICIANS AND SCIENTISTS IN THE U.S.

263 CONCLUDING REMARKS

PREFACE

Imagine that you're in the emergency room of a hospital in a foreign country. You have severe stomach pain and a fever. Was it something you ate? Or is it something more serious? The doctor is trying to help but doesn't speak your language or understand a word you're saying. You're so sick that even speaking a few words is difficult. The family member with you doesn't speak the doctor's language either and is too emotional and afraid to be of much help. The doctor concludes that it's something you ate and sends you back to your hotel with some pain killers, an antibiotic and instructions to come back if the symptoms persist. You spend the next 24 hours feeling increasingly sick until the pain becomes so unbearable that you decide to go back to the hospital. Fortunately, this time there is a nurse who speaks your language. After running some tests, they rush you into the operating room. You have appendicitis and waiting another minute could be the difference between life and death.

Now imagine that person is your son or your daughter, your mom or your dad, your sister or brother, your husband or wife, your best friend or your neighbor. Imagine that this happened today, that the language you and your loved one speak is Spanish, that as you both rush into the emergency room, he or she is crying: "¡Un doctor, por favor!" (A doctor, please!). Now imagine that the foreign country is your home, the United States of America. Or don't imagine it; simply look at the statistics. Situations in which people with low English proficiency are unable to communicate with healthcare providers occur every single day all around a nation where the diversity of the population does not match the diversity of the healthcare workforce.

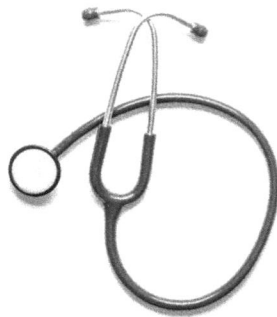

The internet is full of stories [1-4] like that of Gricelda, a 13-year-old girl whose Spanish-speaking parents took her to the hospital because of severe abdominal pain. She was diagnosed with gastritis and sent home, only to die of a perforated appendix a couple of days later. Or Willie, an 18-year-old athlete who was diagnosed with a drug overdose because of a misinterpretation of the word intoxicado (meaning food poisoning in Spanish) and ended up quadriplegic because he was actually having a brain hemorrhage. Or Mrs. Jimenez, who suffered irreversible brain damage while her English-speaking daughter was on the phone attempting to translate for the emergency room physician. Or the 7-year-old who was taken by his Spanish-speaking parents to a pediatrician for weeks only to go into multi-organ failure before the incorrect strep diagnosis was recognized to correspond to Kawasaki's disease. [4, 5]

Some people will say that these highly publicized cases are rare, that they are in the media because they were tragic, and that focusing on them fails to acknowledge the thousands of Spanish-speaking patients who receive culturally and linguistically appropriate care in the United States.

I say our goal as a nation should be to prevent these tragic miscommunications from happening, ever. No one, regardless of their race or ethnicity should die or receive inappropriate care of any kind because of their inability to communicate with their health care provider. Each of these cases represents a human life that could have been saved—a sister, a brother, a friend, a father, a mother—a life that meant everything to their close ones. I urge you to consider the fact that every day, due to an inability to properly communicate, hundreds of people experience situations that even if not life-threatening deeply affect their physical and emotional well-being, their quality of life.

It's been said that "details create the big picture." These individual stories are important because they allow us to put faces to the statistics. They allow us to go from large, nationwide numbers to stories that real people like you and I experience every day.

Patients who have difficulty communicating with their healthcare providers are less able to follow discharge instructions provided in English. They are less adherent to treatment because they don't understand the importance of taking their medicines as directed. And they are less likely to come back for a follow-up visit knowing that they won't be understood. These patients feel disrespected and powerless. Needless to say, this communication gap also deeply affects the ability of practicing physicians—who cannot possibly speak as many languages as the patients they encounter—to appropriately address medical needs to the best of their ability.

The Hispanic population is the largest and the fastest growing minority in the U.S. [6] Other than English, Spanish is the most commonly spoken language. In fact, as many as 40 million U.S. residents age 5 and older speak Spanish at home and more than 16 million households report speaking English "less than very well." Forty million people speaking Spanish at home in the United States is likely an underestimation because many Spanish-speaking residents and immigrants do not participate in the U.S. Census and thus are not counted. [7-10]

To make matters worse, our complex healthcare system is difficult to navigate even for native English speakers. In addition, Hispanics have the lowest levels of health literacy.

I have spent all of my adult life in science and medicine in different capacities, and I have rarely, if ever, worked with another Hispanic physician in the U.S. It is a well-known fact that the racial composition of the nation's physician workforce differs from that of the general population. Numerous articles and books have been written on this topic. However, even though the information is abundant it is also incredibly scattered, difficult to find and even more difficult to interpret, particularly for those of us who are not experts on these topics.

This book is an attempt to understand why there's such lack of diversity in the healthcare workforce, when the disparities begin, how this lack of diversity impacts health outcomes among Hispanics, and whether the problem can be solved with more education among physicians of all races and ethnicities on culturally and linguistically competent care. This book is simply an effort to share what I have learned. My objective was to put it all together in a way that would allow more us to see the big picture and get the conversation going. By addressing some of these questions simply and clearly, I hope to broaden our understanding of this problem so that we can find solutions.

I begin the book by describing the current demographic characteristics of the Hispanic population in the U.S. I am not a demographer, a sociologist or a statistician. Therefore, I may be accused of oversimplifying. However, even a general understanding the data helps raise our awareness of the current state of the Hispanic population in terms of educational attainment and health outcomes. My goal for this book is to go "beyond the numbers" and help readers recognize that culturally and linguistically competent health care providers can make a positive difference in the health outcomes of the Hispanic population in the U.S.

As we go through the different chapters, I share the story of a girl named Ana Maria, who was one of the strongest inspirations for me to go through the journey of writing this book. Ana Maria is a real person I met online and whose name I have modified to respect her privacy. I wanted to learn more about young Hispanics interested in careers in medicine in the U.S. and began reading social media posts. When I read Ana Maria's post saying that her counselor told her that she was not "college material," I almost broke into tears of anger and indignation to learn that a school counselor can say something like that to a young girl with such great aspirations.

Shortly after I started writing this book, I read Michelle Obama's book Becoming. In her book she describes the exact same experience of being told by her school counselor that she was "not Princeton material." Reading that paragraph made me realize that this is a common issue and since then I've heard the same thing multiple times. I decided to share Ana Maria's story in order to help bring the numbers and statistics presented throughout the book to life and to give them meaning.

Despite these sobering facts, this book does not present a gloomy picture of the status of health or education among Hispanics. On the contrary, my research revealed a wonderful truth: we've made remarkable progress. The Hispanic population lags behind other races and ethnicities in most measures. However, when looking at the data over time, the number of Hispanics obtaining a bachelor's degree has doubled in the last decade, and there are more Hispanics going to college and more than ever going to medical school. The future is bright and "¡Si se puede!" (Yes we can!) get to a point where at least there are as many Hispanics in health care as there are individuals of any other race or ethnicity.

Last but not least, the part of the book I'm most proud of and grateful for celebrates contributions from Hispanic physicians in the U.S. who are focused on giving back to the Hispanic community. I strongly believe that it is our moral responsibility as successful Hispanics to serve as mentors. I will forever be grateful to these physicians for their willingness to share their stories with me, and through me with you all. Like the girl on the book cover, I hope reading about them encourages you to see yourself as one of many next-generation Hispanic physicians and heroes. I sincerely hope reading about them makes you all realize that even if the journey is long and difficult, if you persevere and believe in the importance of giving back, then ¡Yes you can!

Why choose this book?

Many authors have written about this topic, but the information is directed to educators, researchers and policy makers. I could not identify books for the general public that compiled all the information and presented it in a concise manner. My first realization upon embarking on the journey of writing this book was that unless you are a demographer or a statistician, it is incredibly difficult to interpret the vast amounts of available data. This explains why I, along with most of the Hispanic and non-Hispanic people I spoke to during the course of writing this book, was unaware of many key pieces of information. For example, most people I spoke with did not know how we—Latin American and Spanish-speaking people—are counted in the census, what the census data is used for, how many Hispanics live in the U.S., and what percentage of them are physicians. Most could not articulate the reasons behind the shortage of Hispanic physicians in the U.S., attributing it almost exclusively to the high cost of tuition, and they did not know the meaning of terms such as "health literacy," "cultural competence" or "determinants of health."

Unless Hispanics understand who we are, how many, what unites us, and what our needs are, not only as individuals but as a group; it will be difficult to fight against inequality. Unless we understand the relevance of our numbers and participate in the census, how can we expect that our needs will be met? As a community, we share the responsibility of addressing the issue of inequality with the government and other public and private institutions.

How to use this book?

The healthcare needs of a population cannot be measured or met without knowledge of the size and characteristics of that population. Therefore, it is not possible to make a case for increased diversity in medicine without defining and describing the Hispanic population. This is why I have chosen to first present the numbers and then go beyond the numbers to talk about the needs.

As shown below, the book is divided in three sections with two chapters per section. Each chapter pair summarizes the demographic data relevant to each topic and is followed by a description of what that information means. The final section contains the personal stories of Hispanic physicians practicing in the U.S.

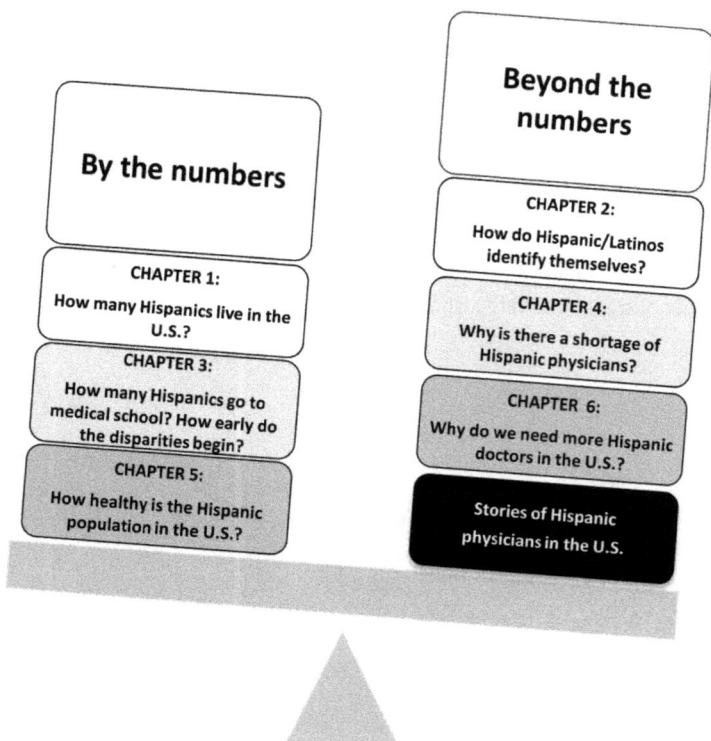

By the numbers

Beyond the numbers

CHAPTER 1:
How many Hispanics live in the U.S.?

CHAPTER 2:
How do Hispanic/Latinos identify themselves?

CHAPTER 3:
How many Hispanics go to medical school? How early do the disparities begin?

CHAPTER 4:
Why is there a shortage of Hispanic physicians?

CHAPTER 5:
How healthy is the Hispanic population in the U.S.?

CHAPTER 6:
Why do we need more Hispanic doctors in the U.S.?

Stories of Hispanic physicians in the U.S.

Additional resources

Online resources: If you are interested in learning more about any of the topics, go to this section for addresses to websites used in each chapter. The e-book version of this title contains direct links to all resources that can be accessed from your computer and other electronic devices.

Key takeaways: If you are only interested in the key conclusions from the chapter, simply go to the key takeaways section that summarizes the entire chapter in a few bullet points.

Infographics: All sections that refer to statistical data have been complemented with more than 50 graphs to make the information easier to understand. For quick access to the graphs just go to the table of figures at the end of the book.

References: Almost all statements related to the status of the Hispanic population in terms of demographics, risk factors for educational attainment or Hispanic identity are thoroughly referenced. I have included more than 300 references for those interested in learning more about any of the topics.

Glossary: One of the most difficult aspects when reading demographic data is the terminology. For that reason I have included a glossary that provides definitions to commonly used terms.

Ana Maria's story: Each section of the book is introduced by part of Ana Maria's story. Even if you don't read the information within each chapter, I encourage you to read her story and share it with others interested in helping the Hispanic community thrive. Please remind Ana Maria and all other students like her not to listen to naysayers. Our answer to them should always be "Yes, we can!" "¡Si se puede!"

HISPANIC/ LATINO IDENTITY

"What makes someone American isn't just blood or birth but allegiance to our founding principles and faith in the idea that anyone -from anywhere- can write the next chapter of our story."
– President Barack Obama

ANA MARIA'S STORY

I met Ana Maria online. In her first social media post, she shared a conversation she had with her high school counselor.

Ana Maria recalls, "Once, I arrived fifteen minutes late for a meeting with my counselor. I politely knocked on the door and the counselor invited me in:

"'You are late, Ana Maria!' the counselor said. 'You do realize that I am a busy person that needs to see other students, right?'

"I apologized, explaining, 'My sister is at the hospital and I needed to help. As you know, my parents don't speak English, and someone had to explain to the doctor what happened to my sister after she missed her second insulin injection last night. My parents can't afford it. They kept us waiting for a doctor for a very long time.'

"Ok, alright," the counselor replied. "What can I do for you?"

"My hands started shaking. I had spent the last few weeks thinking about what I would do after graduation, and even though I had heard a million times from my father that they didn't have enough money to put me through college, I had always dreamt of becoming a doctor.

I wanted to help people like my sister Sofia who was diagnosed with diabetes when she was only six-years-old. I really poured my heart out in front of the counselor.

"The counselor interrupted my story and spoke bluntly. 'Ana Maria, let me stop you right there. I don't mean to crush your dreams, but I honestly don't think you are college material. College is expensive, and with your grades, I'm not sure you will be able to get financial aid,' The counselor paused for a moment, then continued, 'Not to mention your complicated situation at home. How many times have you been late or missed school because you were taking care of your younger siblings? I just can't see this working, Ana Maria. I am sorry.'

"I got up, feeling the weight of the world on my shoulders. I ran out of the office sobbing. I remember the sadness I felt that day and how foolish it all seemed to even think that the counselor would be able to provide a solution. I had a 5-year-old brother waiting for me after school, and an apartment to tidy up before Sofia came back home from the hospital. My mother was working two jobs to help my father, who is a construction worker, pay for the hospital bills for my sister that were piling up. I felt like there would be no end to this struggle."

Sadly, Ana Maria represents thousands of young Hispanics who are told that pursuing a career in medicine is not even an option for them.

CHAPTER ONE

HISPANICS
BY THE
NUMBERS

Counting Hispanics in the U.S.

"... a community of limitless diversity connected by one ethnicity
– proof that identity is far from skin deep. Latinos don't fit into a
census box, a stereotype or a mold. Latinos break the mold."
- The Huffington Post, Latinos Break the Mold Initiative

The terminology: Hispanic, Latino, Latina, Latinx

The term "Latino" may be understood as shorthand for the Spanish word "Latinoamericano" (Latin American). It is rarely used outside of the United States where the demonym corresponding to the country of origin is preferred, e.g. Mexican, Ecuadorian, Colombian, etc.

Dictionaries define a Latin person as a native or inhabitant of Latin America (South America, Central America or Mexico), or a person of Latin American origin who lives in the United States. [11]

The feminine adjective Latina became prevalent in the 1970s when feminist movements pushed for gender recognition among Latinos in the United States. Most recently, the gender-neutral alternative Latinx, which was introduced to the Merriam-Webster dictionary in 2018, has gained popularity in the media. [12]

The term "Hispanic" is typically associated to the use of the Spanish language. The word came into existence in the mid-1500s and is defined as "of, or relating to the people, speech, or culture of Spain." [13]

In contemporary usage, some of the official definitions of the term Hispanic include:
1. Someone "relating to Spain or to Spanish-speaking countries, especially those of Central and South America" [11]
2. Someone who is "of, relating to, or being a person of Latin American descent and especially of Cuban, Mexican, or Puerto Rican origin living in the U.S." [13]
3. Someone coming originally from an area where Spanish is spoken and especially from Latin America." [14]

The terms Hispanic and Latino are often used interchangeably. Even though both terms are used for people who live in the United States, the key distinction between them according to most definitions, is the association of the adjective Hispanic with the use of the Spanish language, and Latino with the use of all Latin-based Romance languages as well as with the geographic origin of the person or his/her ancestry. In fact, the term Latino includes people from Brazil where Portuguese, not Spanish, is the official language.

As we will discuss in the next section, the U.S. Census Bureau uses three terms in the census questionnaire: Hispanic/Latino/Spanish origin.

The controversy

Deciding on the best terminology to be used in the census in order to accurately count people and appropriately distribute resources aroused much controversy among the members of an advisory committee put in place during the Nixon administration. [15] The committee, which included Mexicans, Puerto Ricans, Cubans and members of other races and ethnicities, [16-18] chose the term "Hispanic" over "Latino."

Opponents of the use of either term say that one word cannot possibly capture the multidimensional and heterogeneous nature of the demographic they represent, that pan-ethnic terms assume that all members of that demographic are the same regardless of their nationality, and that the only reason why these terms were popularized was to make the community more marketable, not because the community identifies with them. [19] The use of the word "Hispanic" has also been criticized for years, primarily because it is considered a nod towards Spanish colonialism.

> *"I hope that my daughter will be conscious that the idea of Latino/ Hispanic was actually rooted in an effort to work for social justice and political inclusion. Though we are a diverse community, many still grapple with disadvantage, discrimination and underrepresentation.*
> *- Cristina Mora, Making Hispanics: how activists, bureaucrats, and media constructed a new American*

> *"Words such as Hispanic or Latino are limiting. We come in all shapes, sizes, colors and dialects. There's no one word that fits all."*
> *– Lawrence Hernandez*

One of the main arguments against the use of the noun "Latinx" is the idea that it would erase the results of the feminist movement that fought to highlight the role and identity of Latin American females in the United States. In 2018, Latinx was officially excluded from the dictionary of the Real Academia Española, which rejects the use of "x" and "e" as gender-neutral alternatives. An argument in its favor relates to the advantages of using gender-neutral, inclusive language, which is why this new word is gaining momentum in social media and among the LGBT community.

Which term do most Hispanic/Latinos prefer?

> *"All in all, I hope my daughter will embrace her Latinidad by being conscious of its roots in social justice and by continuing the cause of civil rights and political participation in America."*
> *– Cristina Mora, Making Hispanics: how activists, bureaucrats, and media constructed a new American*

When surveying large samples of the population, it turns out that only 20% of Hispanics living in the U.S. use the pan-ethnic terms "Hispanic" or "Latino" to describe their identity.[20] In a survey of 5,103 Hispanics from several countries, 50% of participants said that they had no preference between the terms Hispanic or Latino. Among those who do have a preference, 33% said that they prefer the term Hispanic while 15% chose Latino. In spite of some variation due to age and other factors, Hispanic was usually the first choice.[20, 21]

I have chosen to use the term "Hispanic" in this book to be respectful of that choice, and because the importance of Spanish language or linguistically appropriate communication in health care is a key message of this book. However, occasionally I will use the term "Latino" to respect the choice of the authors I am quoting.

Our goal as a community is to remember that patients of all races and ethnicities, including Hispanic/Latino need and deserve fair and appropriate health care. The terms that we use to define each population are used primarily as a way of quantifying the needs of each population, not of defining its true identity.

In the following sections, I will explain how the Hispanic/Latino terminology is used by the U.S. Census Bureau and summarize key demographic characteristics of the Hispanic population using data from the U.S. Census and the American Community Survey (ACS).

Without clear knowledge of the demographics, it is difficult to estimate our needs, such as the sufficiency of the healthcare workforce. Similarly, without good knowledge of how the data is collected; it is difficult to understand why the available data may underestimate those needs.

The United States Census

What is it?

"Census" is a Latin word that was used during the Roman Republic to describe a survey conducted to keep track of all adult males fit for military service. In the United States, our Founding Fathers empowered Congress to conduct a census to count every person living in the country, to determine Congressional representation. The first census took place on August 2, 1790.

What is the information used for?

In addition to enumerating the population, early versions of the U.S. census were also used for taxation and to recruit youth into military service. However, since 1954, it is constitutional to include questions in the census beyond those concerning a simple count of the number of people (13 U.S.C. §141). The ACS is conducted every year to collect information about social and economic needs of the population including education, housing, health care needs, jobs, etc. in order to distribute resources accordingly. This is one of the reasons why participation in the census is so important.

Does Census data accurately represent the Hispanic population?

I will be using census data throughout the book, but it is important to highlight its limitations pertaining to the undercounting of specific populations, particularly Hispanics.

As William P. O'Hare states in the introductory chapter of his book *Differential Undercounts in the U.S. Census: Who is missed?*, "The mantra of the U.S. Census Bureau is to count every person once, only once, and in the right place. This is easy to say, but difficult to achieve." In his book he describes in detail the potential consequences of miscounting minority populations including its impact on the distribution of public funds, political power, public perceptions on population growth, funding of scientific and civil rights programs, among others. His book [22] and several others [8, 10, 23] are great resources for those interested in the topic of population undercounting, especially as it pertains to the 2020 census, as well as for more information about "hard-to-count populations."

In this section, I will briefly summarize four aspects that may be particularly relevant to the issues related to undercounting the Hispanic population:
1. The definitions of race and ethnicity;
2. The increasing number of individuals who do not identify themselves with any of the official race categories in the census questionnaire;
3. The difficulty collecting information among Spanish-speaking individuals and among those who live in remote areas;
4. The recent controversy around collecting citizenship information in the decennial census.

In the next chapter I will explore additional considerations related to Hispanic identity that also influence census counts.

How does the U.S. census collect race and ethnicity data?

In his New York Times opinion article: "The Americans Our Government Won't Count," Alex Wagner states: "Racially speaking, the United States is 0% Hispanic. This is confusing—especially for America's nearly 58 million Hispanics." [7]

The Census Bureau collects racial data in accordance with guidelines provided by the U.S. Office of Management and Budget (OMB). [24]

The current version of the survey examines race and ethnicity with two questions: "Is the person of Hispanic, Latino or Spanish origin?" and "What is this person's race?"

Thus, in the census questionnaire, it is ethnicity that determines whether a person is of Hispanic origin or not. The OMB requires a minimum of two categories in collecting and reporting data. For this reason, ethnicity is broken out in two options, Hispanic or Latino and Not Hispanic or Latino. [24]

The question on Hispanic origin includes five response categories: one for respondents who do not identify as Hispanic and the following four for those who do:
1. "Mexican, Mexican Am., Chicano"
2. "Puerto Rican"
3. "Cuban"
4. "Another Hispanic, Latino, or Spanish origin"

Respondents have a space where they can write a specific Hispanic origin group e.g. Peruvian.

The second, separate question is about race. Hispanics can report any race and, since 2010, all respondents may report more than one race. The U.S. Census Bureau states that "Hispanic origin can be viewed as the heritage, nationality, lineage, or country of birth of the person or the person's parents or ancestors before arriving in the United States. People who identify as Hispanic, Latino, or Spanish may be any race." The OMB requires five minimum categories for race:
1. White
2. Black or African American
3. Asian
4. American Indian and Alaska Native, Native Hawaiian and Other Pacific Islander
5. Some Other Race (SOR)

Respondents have a space where they can write a specific Hispanic origin group.

As shown in Box 1, a separate question about Hispanic origin was not introduced until 1980, and the option to choose more than one race and to enter a specific "group" of Hispanic origin were not introduced until 2000. What this means is that

Hispanics of all nationalities and races were counted together until fairly recently, so we are just beginning to collect information on the true heterogeneity of the Hispanic population. Even with the current version of the census questionnaire, data collection is inaccurate for the reasons discussed next.

BOX 1. WHEN DID HISPANIC IMMIGRATION BEGIN IN THE U.S. AND WHEN DID THE U.S. CENSUS START COUNTING HISPANICS?

Since the passing of the 1965 Immigration and Nationality Act approximately 59 million immigrants have arrived in the United States. In contrast to the immigration waves of the mid and late 1800s, which brought approximately 14 million immigrants to the U.S., almost all European, half of the immigrants coming to the country since 1965 have come from Latin America, and one-quarter from Asia. [25]

The Hispanic population grew faster than any other racial or ethnic group between 1990 and 2013. For example, more than 1 million Hispanics were added to the U.S. population between July 1, 2015, and July 1, 2016. This number is more than half of the approximately 2 million people added to the nation's total population during that period. Even though that growth has slowed down in some parts of the country where Asian Americans are showing a slightly faster growth, other areas like North Dakota have experienced a dramatic growth in the Hispanic population. [26]

The first attempt to enumerate Hispanics appeared as part of the race question, which had a category for "Mexican" in the **1930** census.

The terminology of "Central, South American, Puerto Rican, Cuban, Mexican, Other Spanish" was introduced in **1970**, but the question on Hispanic origin was only included in long-form questionnaires sent to a sample of the population, resulting in severe undercounts.

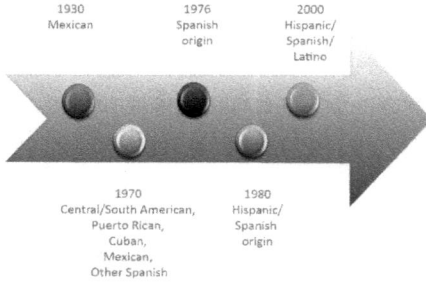

Changes in the race/ethnicity categories used in the U.S. census 1930-present

1930
Mexican

1976
Spanish origin

2000
Hispanic/ Spanish/ Latino

1970
Central/South American, Puerto Rican, Cuban, Mexican, Other Spanish

1980
Hispanic/ Spanish origin

FIGURE 1. CHANGES TO RACE AND ETHNICITY CATEGORIES IN THE U.S. CENSUS OVERTIME

In **1976**, the U.S. Congress passed the only law in this country's history that mandated the collection and analysis of data for a specific ethnic group to determine the urgent and special needs of "Americans of Spanish origin" defined as: "Americans who identify themselves as being of Spanish-speaking background and who trace their origin or descent from Mexico, Puerto Rico, Cuba, Central and South America and other Spanish-speaking countries." [27]

A separate question about Hispanic origin was not introduced until **1980**. [23] The question was "Is this person of Hispanic/Spanish origin or descent?" If the answer was yes, four options were provided (1) Mexican, Mexican American, Chicano, (2) Puerto Rican, (3) Cuban, or (4) other Spanish/ Hispanic.

The **2000** census was the first to introduce the term "Latino." The previous question was replaced by: "Is this person Hispanic/Spanish/Latino? The same four options were provided, but this time those choosing "other Hispanic/Spanish/Latino" had the option to type in a "group" e.g. Colombian, Peruvian. This was also the first census to allow Americans to report a multiracial origin.

The **2010** U.S. Census included changes to more clearly distinguish Hispanic ethnicity as not being a race. In that Census the following sentence was added: "For this census, Hispanic origins are not races."
Until today, the U.S. Census Bureau uses the ethnonym Hispanic or Latino to refer to "a person of Cuban, Mexican, Puerto Rican, South or Central

American, or other Spanish culture or origin regardless of race" and states that Hispanics or Latinos can be of any race, any ancestry, and any ethnicity. Additionally, the terms were modified from "Hispanic or Latino" to "Hispanic, Latino or Spanish origin." Origin refers to the heritage, nationality group, lineage, or country of birth of the person or the person's ancestors before their arrival in the United States.

Some other race?

The overwhelming majority of census respondents choose only one race. However, there is a growing number of individuals in the U.S. who do not identify themselves with any of the official race categories or who consider themselves multiracial. [28] In 2017, more than 15 million (4.8%) respondents chose the Some Other Race option, and more than 10 million (3.1%) chose two or more races. The third most common racial group after White and Asian is "Some Other Race" and it comprises primarily Hispanics. [29]

> *"Are Latino-Americans White? Black? Other? Illegal aliens from Mars? Or are we the very face of America?"*
> *- Raquel Cepeda, Bird of Paradise: How I Became Latina*

Hispanics have great difficulty responding to the race question when presented with separate race and Hispanic origin questions. [30] Approximately 40% of Hispanic respondents chose the "Some Other Race (SOR)" category in the 2000 and 2010 census. [31] For example, there are 3.3 million White people in the Greater Boston area. Over 300,000 of them identify themselves as Latino, and as many as 134,000 of those who identify themselves as Latino report belonging to "Some Other Race." [32-34]

Without a modification in the Census questions, the SOR category could become the second most common "race" in the 2020 census. For this reason, the Bureau conducted the "2010 Census Alternative Questionnaire Experiment (AQE) Research on Race and Hispanic Origin," which was the most comprehensive research effort on race and Hispanic origin ever undertaken. [35] The project proposed a unified race and ethnicity question that treated Hispanic origin as a race, which corresponds to how most Americans think of ethno-racial groups. The unified question led to a dramatic reduction to 0.2% in the number of Americans (mostly Hispanic) who claim an SOR option on race. Consequently, the percentage of people reporting White race also decreased.

The bureau conducted the 2015 National content test in 1.2 million U.S. households, 45% of which identified themselves as Hispanic. [36] In this test, Hispanic origin and race were combined into one question. More than 70% Hispanics responded "Hispanic" but did not choose any other race. In contrast, when asked separately one third checked SOR and one third checked two or more races.

Unfortunately, in spite of these results, it has already been announced by the current administration that the 2020 census will not combine the race and Hispanic origin questions. This much needed change in the way data is collected is likely to be reintroduced for approval under a future presidential administration.

Many people fear that this issue contradicts the way Hispanics think about themselves and that it will affect projections about Hispanic population needs. In a written statement, Arturo Vargas, executive director of the National Association of Latino Elected and Appointed Officials Educational Fund, said that the decision ignores years of research and the expert advice of scientists.

One of the implications of these findings, for our discussion, is that Hispanics who speak Spanish or live in households where Spanish is the primary language and maintain deeply rooted cultural connections with their Hispanic ancestry and traditions, do consider culturally appropriate health care to be critically important. On the contrary, those members of the Hispanic community who do not identify themselves as Hispanics or do not live in households where Spanish is the primary language may see no advantage in being treated by a Hispanic physician, and may not understand the importance of culturally appropriate health care. I will talk about Hispanic identity in the next chapter, to clarify how many Hispanics are estimated to fall in each of these categories and how they are distinct.

Language and surveying rural areas

Language barriers increase the risk that U.S. residents with limited English proficiency are not adequately counted in the census. This issue can only be addressed if most Hispanics with limited English proficiency receive a bilingual form. The U.S. Census Bureau determines language use and speaking ability though essentially three questions:

1. Does this person speak a language other than English at home? Yes or no?
2. What is this language?
3. How well does this person speak English? "Very well," "Well," "Not well," or "Not at all." This is based on the respondent's own perception about his or her own ability, or the perception of another household member responding to the survey.

In an effort to increase the participation of minorities and marginalized communities, data from the ACS is analyzed yearly to estimate the number of limited-English speaking households in the U.S., and to determine which languages to include in census instruction translations. Even though there is a significantly lower undercount in areas receiving bilingual questionnaires, research has shown that the difference is small. **The 2010 Census was the first one to use a bilingual English/Spanish questionnaire, but unfortunately only half (46%) of all Hispanics lived in areas that received bilingual questionnaires.**
For the 2020 census, the U.S. Census Bureau plans to provide the Internet Self-Response Instrument and Census Questionnaire Assistance in 12 non-English languages. The paper census forms are available in Spanish and English. [37]

"The purpose of the census isn't to count citizens, but to count people."
- The Times Editorial Board, Los Angeles Times, Jan 4, 2018

In 2019, the Supreme Court ruled against a question on citizenship to be included in the 2020 Census. Proponents of this change still argue that this question is critical to understanding the population of eligible voters in order to prevent racial discrimination at the polls. Detractors argue that such a change is costly and would produce less accurate data. Also, given the current political environment, many believe that there is a political underpinning in the recommendation of the current administration to include citizenship information in the census, and that the best way to undermine the strength in our numbers is to refuse to accurately count Hispanics in the first place. However, as Alex Wagner says in his New York Times article, in an environment in which "whiteness" gives people a sense of belonging, to self-identify as Hispanic or Arabic-American is a political act. [7]

Even though the Census Bureau adheres to confidentiality laws that prohibit sharing of respondent information with tax collection agencies and law enforcement and immigration services, asking people about their citizenship status is likely to lead illegal immigrants to avoid participating in the census for fear of deportation.

Research from the Urban Institute has already suggested that even though the court ruled against the question on citizenship, the public attention to the topic has generated enough concern among immigrants that they are less likely to participate in the 2020 census regardless. In a recent study, researchers from Harvard Kennedy School asked approximately 9,000 people to fill out a questionnaire with questions taken verbatim from the U.S. Census survey. Half of the respondents were asked: "Is this person a citizen of the United States?" Asking about citizenship status significantly increased the number of questions skipped. The strongest effects were observed among Hispanics who were less likely to report having Hispanic household members. The researchers extrapolated these numbers to the national level and estimated that the inclusion of a citizensh p question in the census would result in an undercounting of approximately 6 million Hispanics in the 2020 Census. Even though there are several caveats associated with this study, which the authors point out in their publication, it is not counterintuitive to assume that a question on citizenship could result in undercounting. This is simply one of the few scientific studies to confirm that assumption. [8, 38]

Of note, the citizenship question is already being asked every year to a subset of the population as part of the ACS. In the 2017 survey, the question on citizenship went unanswered by 1 in 12 Hispanics. Hispanics from Mexico and Central America were among the groups most likely to skip the question, suggesting that they would be at highest risk of undercounting if the citizenship question was ever added to the census. [39]

Using tabulations from the ACS, the Pew Research Center has reported that the majority of Hispanics living in the United States are U.S. citizens by birth or naturalization (79%). However, this number includes Puerto Ricans, who are virtually all U.S. Citizens, and Spaniards, Panamanians and Mexicans who have high citizenship rates of 91, 89 and 79%, respectively. The percentage of citizens varies among all other nationalities of origin. About half of Venezuelans, Guatemalans and Hondurans in the U.S. are citizens and only about 7 in 10 Hispanics of all other nationalities have U.S. citizenship. It is estimated that in 2016, about 34% of Hispanics in the United States were foreign-born with only 12% of those having citizenship.

Participation in the census allows us to make a statement to clarify who we really are. Some efforts are taking place to provide education around the census questionnaire and the immense implications of the results on the allocation of resources, which many Hispanics are not aware of. For all communities to get their fair share of public funds for programs including those involving education and health care, participation in the Census is vital.

"We must be impatient for change. Let us remember that our voice is a precious gift and we must use it."
- Claudia Flores, Associate Clinical Professor of Law, Director, International Human Rights Clinic

How many Hispanics are currently in the U.S.?

By July of 2018, the total population of the United States was 325.7 million. [29] Of those, 59.9 million (18%) were Hispanic or Latino of any race, making the Hispanic population the largest minority in the United States.

Of the more than 59 million Hispanics, 36.6 million were Mexican, 5.58 Puerto Rican, 2.3 Cuban, and 14.3 million were categorized as Other Hispanic or Latino.

A great percentage of the Hispanic population concentrates in certain regions of the country. Nine U.S. states have a population of at least 1 million Hispanics: Arizona, California, Colorado, Florida, Illinois, New Jersey, New Mexico, New York and Texas, with California having the largest Hispanic population in the country.

Will the Hispanic population be larger than the white population in the near future?

The expectation that the number of Hispanics in the U.S. will increase to 119 million by 2060, and that Non-Hispanic whites will become less than half of the U.S. population by 2055 has been broadly publicized in recent years. This estimation is based on data from the U.S. Census, and it does have some caveats.

First, it depends on counting all children of mixed-race families as non-White, which some people consider inappropriate, as these children do not think of themselves as part of a minority [34] (see also the section on Hispanic racial identity). This is important because as many as one of every seven infants comes from an ethno-racially mixed family and because since 2015, more than half of all babies in the United States are born into a racial or ethnic minority family. [40] However, some people argue that to count people of Hispanic heritage as White is also inappropriate. This is likely to occur as well, because half of fourth-generation Hispanics do not identify themselves as Hispanic, [41] highlighting the importance of self-identity trends in the final counts.

As discussed earlier in this chapter, another important argument to consider is the counting of people who choose the "Some Other Race" category. The current two-question (race and ethnicity) format included in the census survey likely undercounts the number of White people who may, in fact, be Hispanics that identify themselves as White (see also the section on Hispanic racial identity). Combining the race and ethnicity questions could result in a decrease in the number of Whites in the U.S.

Key takeaways from chapter 1

1

Only 20% of Hispanics use the controversial terms Hispanic and/or Latino, and the majority of them use the demonym corresponding to their country of origin e.g. Ecuadorian. Those who have a preference, choose "Hispanic," which is a term introduced in the 1970s by an advisory committee trying to identify the best way to describe this population in order to appropriately quantify its needs. Neither term accurately represents the heterogeneity of this population.

2

In the U.S. Census it is ethnicity that determines whether a person is of Hispanic origin or not. Race information is collected separately, and Hispanics can report any race. There are five different race categories: White, Black or African American, Asian, American Indian and Alaska Native, Native Hawaiian and Other Pacific Islander, and Some Other Race (SOR). Many Hispanics choose SOR.

3

The Census does not accurately enumerate the Hispanic population due to several issues including the availability of questionnaires in Spanish in all areas where Spanish-speaking individuals live, the difficulties surveying remote areas, and the confusion around definitions of race and ethnicity. Additionally, a chilling effect from the publicity around the possible addition of a citizenship question could prevent as many as 6 million Hispanics from participating in the 2020 census, even though the question will not be included as ruled by the U.S. Supreme Court.

4

In 2019 there were more than 59.9 million Hispanics in the U.S. corresponding to 18% of the population and making Hispanics the largest minority in the United States. The expectation is that this number will increase to 119 million by 2060.

5

Participation in the census is important. Data from the census is used to determine the distribution of public funds for numerous programs including those involving education and health care.

Online resources for chapter 1

| IF YOU ARE INTERESTED IN: | GO TO: |

| --- | --- |
Accessing data from the decennial census and the ACS	U.S. CENSUS https://www.census.gov/topics/ population/hispanic-origin/about. html The American Community Survey (ACS) is an annual survey that provides information on 46 topics, including income/poverty, employment status, and education level.
Population Projections by race and ethnicity	Population projections out to 2060 are provided by race and Hispanic origin for the nation.
National-level data on the social, economic, and demographic characteristics of selected race groups	The Current Population Survey (CPS) Hispanic Research Center http://www.hispanicresearchcenter. org/publications/the-early-home- environment-of-latino-children-a- research-synthesis/
Data on children and families	Kids Count KIDS COUNT Data Book https://datacenter.kidscount.org/

CHAPTER TWO

HISPANICS BEYOND THE NUMBERS

Hispanic Racial Identity is multidimensional

*"Labels, like Spanish or Hispanic or Latin, come and go,
but identity is something totally separate.
What matters is who I am."*
-Sara Inés Calderón

ANA MARIA DOES NOT IDENTIFY HERSELF AS LATINA, BUT AS MEXICAN

Ana Maria came to the United States when she was nine.

"It is all a bit blurry, but I still remember my mother's tears when she told us that we had to move to the U.S," she recalls.

She grew up in Puebla, Mexico. She still remembers walking to her grandmother's house for lunch every day after school. "*Abuelita* (grandma) had fruit trees in her backyard and she would let me go back there and grab a few if I ate all my food. Fruit was our dessert."

Ana Maria's emotional connection with her home country is strong. Her mom calls Abuelita at least once a week and even though they have not been back to Mexico since they left because the money has been so tight, they send as much as they can every month to Abuelita and Tia (aunt) Susana. "Abuelita is always telling me that I will one day achieve my dream of becoming a doctor. I just don't know how."

It hurts Ana Maria's mother to see her child grow apart from their culture. "Ever since an early age Ana Maria had to adapt, learning the language, the habits – it is all part of her lifestyle now."

Ana Maria says that her mother was always keen to remind her of their country of origin. "She insisted that at home only Spanish will be spoken, unless we have visitors." Family dinners, traditions and holidays, as well as the music and cuisine also remain as an integral part of their lives. Ana Maria talks about how it all was before this big change. "Things seemed so simple. No boundaries or definitions – just people."

If you ask Ana Maria to tell you about herself, she starts by saying "I am Mexican." Her brother, Marco on the other hand, identifies himself as an American. He was born in the U.S., so his ties with Mexico are not as strong as hers. Thanks to federal funding that helps states provide childcare assistance to low-income families, Marco went to a daycare where several caregivers were bilingual, and he's now fluent in English. He has never been to Mexico and, compared to his older sister's, his Spanish proficiency is limited. In spite of his parents' disapproval, Marco usually responds in English when spoken to in Spanish at home.

When asked whether he is embarrassed of his origins, Marco lowers his head, clenches his jaw and states defiantly: "It's not that I'm embarrassed; I was born in the U.S. I am an American!"

"I'm sorry," his mother quickly interjects apologetically. "He just wants to fit in so bad. You know, *niños*."

What is race?

People understand race and ethnicity differently, and as we saw in the previous chapter, this causes confusion when answering census questionnaires and can lead to inaccurate counts. Most people think of "race" as a group of common inborn biological traits (e.g., skin color, shape of the face or nose, color of the eyes or hair,

"I guess it all depends on whom you ask and when you ask. Race, I've learned, is in the eye of the beholder."
- Raquel Cepeda, Bird of Paradise: How I Became Latina

among others). However, there are no biological characteristics that permit the division of each race into a purely distinct category. In fact, although highly debated [42-46], it has been reported that there is more genetic variation within a racial group than across racial groups and thus the existence of unambiguous and perfectly demarcated races and the use of the term "race" are in principle not possible to substantiate with scientific facts.

I leave it to you to make your own judgment, but I personally agree with the following "American Anthropological Association Statement on 'Race'": *"Given what we know about the capacity of normal humans to achieve and function within any culture, we conclude that present-day inequalities between so-called 'racial' groups are not consequences of their biological inheritance but products of historical and contemporary social, economic, educational, and political circumstances."* [47]

The OMB states: *"The racial and ethnic categories set forth in the standards should not be interpreted as being primarily biological or genetic in reference." Race and ethnicity may be thought of in terms of social and cultural characteristics, as well as ancestry,"* [24]

This inclusion is important because of the proposition of a new definition of race in which a complex combination of culture, family traditions, spoken languages, gender identity, and many other factors define who we are beyond our place of birth or that of our ancestors. In fact, many anthropologists and social scientists consider "race" as one of many categories used by societies to divide their members; and others choose to use the word ethnicity, instead of race, to refer to self-identified characteristics that individuals choose themselves instead of being imposed on them. [48]

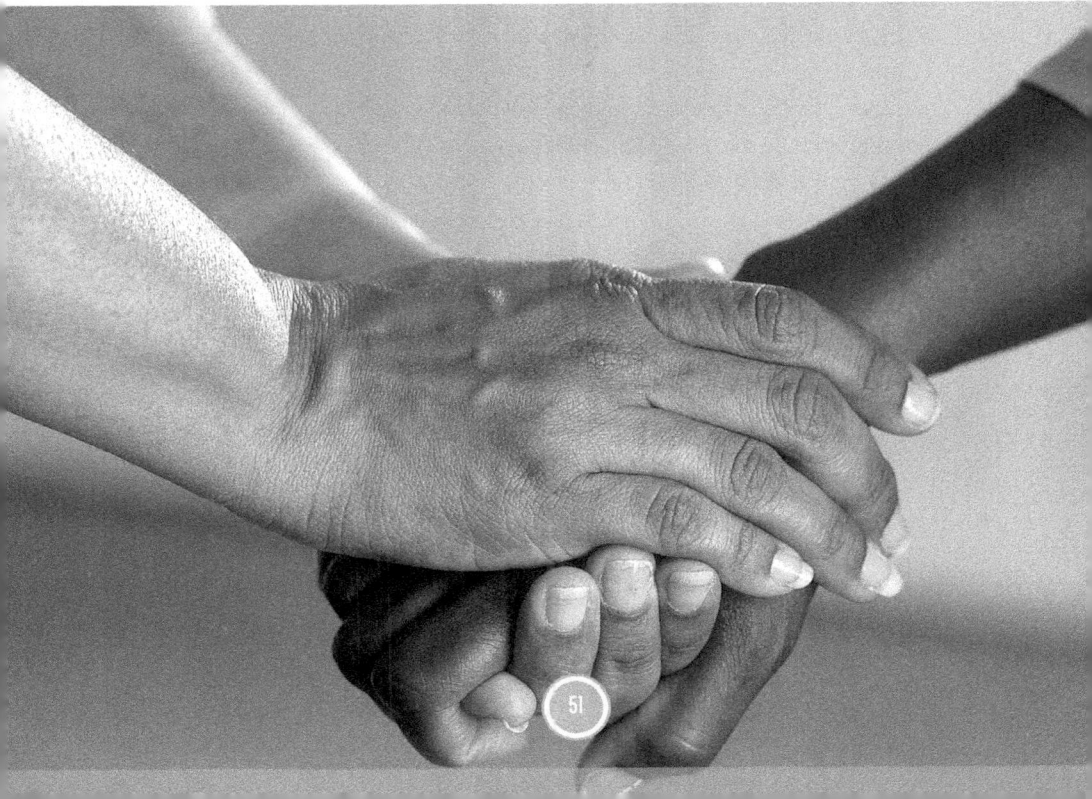

Factors that influence Hispanic racial identity

Racial identity is a complex topic and entire volumes have been written about it. As mentioned before, this book attempts to summarize and simplify complex topics. For that reason, I will only focus on what people like you and I think about racial identity, instead of the more formal or philosophical definition of racial identity as described by others. [49-51]

Using data from the Boundaries in the American Mosaic Survey, investigators analyzed how participants describe their own racial identity when not constrained by fixed definitions such as those used by the census. Those who identified as Hispanic in the initial fixed-choice question were more likely than White and Black respondents to provide what can be termed "nonstandard answers," with many choosing Latino or Latina, but many others choosing either their country of origin or multiple races to define their identity. Even more complexity is revealed in participants' answers when including a follow-up open-ended ethnicity question. [52]

Over the last decade there have been several surveys on how Hispanics/Latinos self-identity. One NBC Latino survey from 2012 showed that as many as three-quarters of Latinos identify themselves as Americans.

Multiple factors influence racial identity. The data summarized below comes primarily from the study on Multiracial America as well as from National Surveys of Latinos conducted by the Pew Research Center. [53, 54] Even though I do not think that this type of research can be generalized to the entire population of Hispanics in the United States, these studies have a sound research design and take into account the way respondents identify themselves. I strongly recommend reading the full reports as they provide interesting insights into Hispanic racial identity. In particular, they demonstrate that there are multiple subgroups among the Hispanic population and thus counting all Hispanic/Latinos together fails to take those factors into account and misrepresents the needs of a heterogeneous population.

SOME OF THE FACTORS THAT INFLUENCE RACIAL IDENTITY

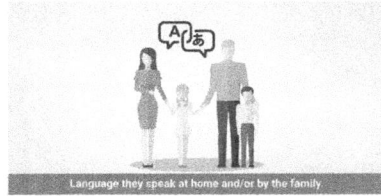

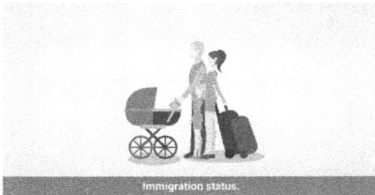

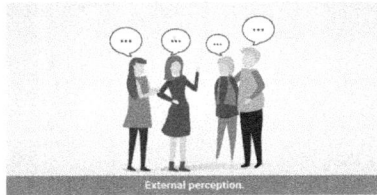

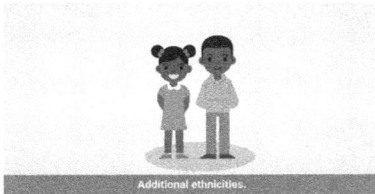

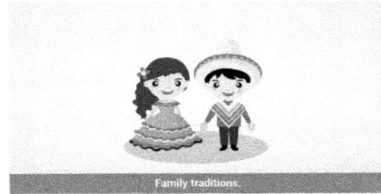

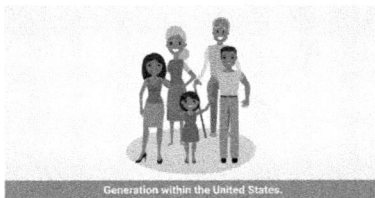

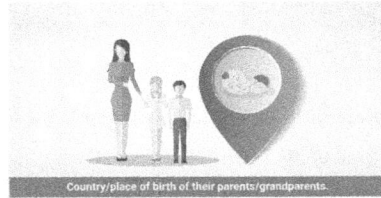

Language they speak at home and/or by the family.

Immigration status.

External perception.

Additional ethnicities.

Family traditions.

Generation within the United States.

Country/place of birth of their parents/grandparents.

FIGURE 2. SOME OF THE MANY FACTORS THAT INFLUENCE RACIAL IDENTITY.

Generation within the United States

The length of time that a person has lived in the United States after immigrating, has a profound impact in all aspects of Hispanic identity, as I will summarize in the next few paragraphs.

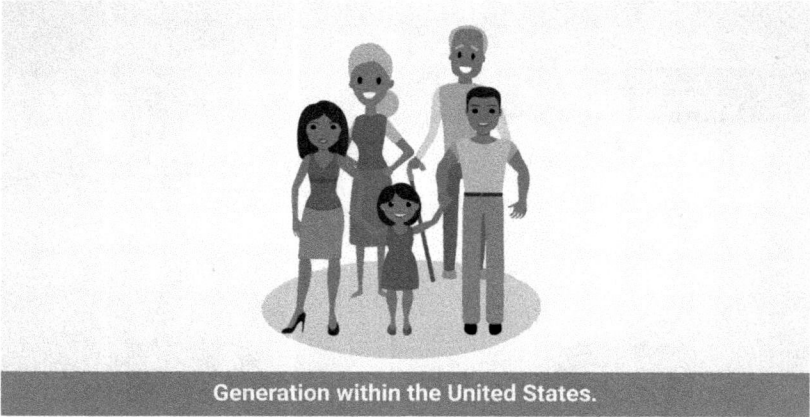

Generation within the United States.

FIGURE 3. FACTORS THAT INFLUENCE HISPANIC IDENTITY: GENERATION WITHIN THE U.S.

Using data from the 2015 Survey of Latinos, Lopez et al. report that the closer they are to their immigrant roots, the more likely Hispanics are to identify themselves as Hispanic. [55] U.S.-born Hispanics, especially third- and fourth-generation, are less likely to identify themselves as Hispanics. [41]

> *I struggled with being a Latina growing up in Los Angeles. I felt very American. I still do. I went to 35 bar mitzvahs before I went to a single quinceanera. I could talk all day about my culture and what it means to me.*
> *– America Ferrera*

Moreover, third-generation or higher respondents are less likely to have participated in Hispanic cultural events, and less likely to say that their parents often talked about feeling proud of their origins. They were also less likely to have been encouraged to speak Spanish or have strong connections with family abroad. The longer they have lived in the United States, the less likely they are to have close Hispanic friends.

Hispanic Identity across Generations

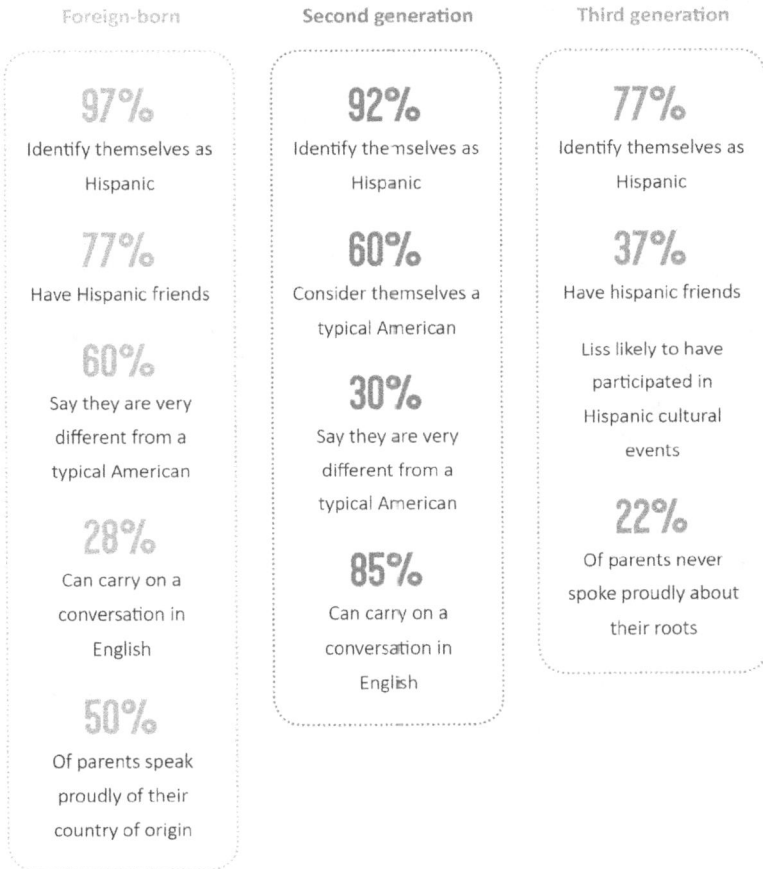

Foreign-born	Second generation	Third generation
97% Identify themselves as Hispanic	**92%** Identify themselves as Hispanic	**77%** Identify themselves as Hispanic
77% Have Hispanic friends	**60%** Consider themselves a typical American	**37%** Have hispanic friends
60% Say they are very different from a typical American	**30%** Say they are very different from a typical American	Liss likely to have participated in Hispanic cultural events
28% Can carry on a conversation in English	**85%** Can carry on a conversation in English	**22%** Of parents never spoke proudly about their roots
50% Of parents speak proudly of their country of origin		

FIGURE 4. FACTORS THAT INFLUENCE HISPANIC IDENTITY ACROSS GENERATIONS

Twice as many second-generation Hispanics said that they consider themselves a "typical American" compared to first-generation Hispanics. Although 60% of first-generation Hispanics responded that they consider themselves "very different from a typical American," this is related to the finding that fewer of them can carry on a conversation in English, while most of second-generation Hispanics can (85%). [56] While almost 6 out of 10 Hispanics who are foreign-born reported participating in cultural celebrations when growing up, only 3 out of 10 of third-generation

Hispanics do. When asked about their connection with their country of origin, as many as 82% of foreign-born Hispanics reported feeling very/somewhat connected to their country of origin. That number decreases to 62% and 49% among second- and third-generation Hispanics, respectively. [41]

First-generation Hispanics and their parents struggle to "fit-in," and suffer discrimination and a sense of being neither "Hispanic enough," nor "American enough." An interesting movement called Project Eñye has been launched recently in the U.S. to tell the story of first-generation Hispanics and their struggle. The name of the movement refers to the pronunciation of the letter ñ. According to their website, the Eñye Nation is a community that helps people "overcome the belief that you are not Latino enough or American enough so you can reawaken the powerful Latino within you and slay in every area of your life by embracing your Latinidad instead of going it alone." Their short documentary film Being ñ is a great illustration of what Hispanic identity means for U.S.-born Latinos.

External perception

Because we are talking about an ethnic group living in a country as a minority, external perception is an important factor influencing racial identity. The way Hispanics feel they are perceived by others varies according to their own perceived racial identity.

"One of the greatest things you have in life is that no one has the authority to tell you what you want to be. You're the one who'll decide what you want to be. Respect yourself and respect the integrity of others as well. The greatest thing you have is your self-image, a positive opinion of yourself. You must never let anyone take it from you."
- Jaime Escalante

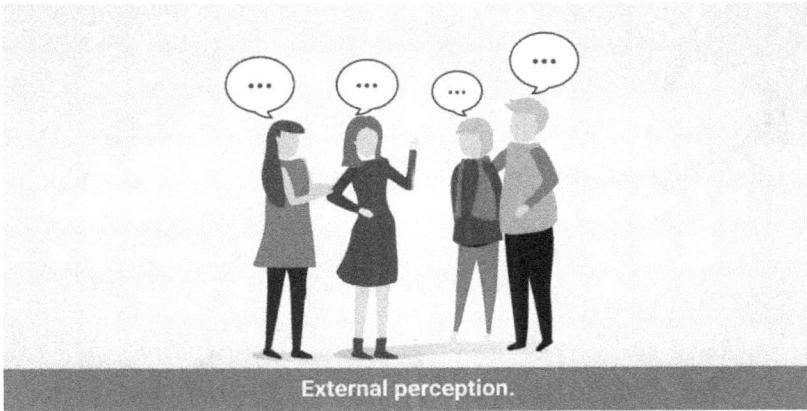

External perception.

FIGURE 5. FACTORS THAT INFLUENCE HISPANIC IDENTITY: EXTERNAL PERCEPTION

As background and to explain the research presented below, the data comes from a survey that used two ways to define racial identity among Hispanics. First, there was a group of respondents (n=261) who said that their racial background includes two or more races, regardless of whether they saw their Hispanic background as a race. [57] For simplicity, I will herein refer to this group as "Two or More Races."

Second, there was a group (n=139) that identified their Hispanic background as their race and who selected one additional census race option, most commonly White. This group will be referred to herein as "Hispanic White." Figure 6 summarizes the key findings of this study.

More "Hispanic White" individuals say that people passing them on the street would think that they're White. Importantly, among Hispanic Whites who choose Hispanic as their race, almost half say that people would think they are Hispanic if they passed them on the street. In the two or more races group 17% of respondents say that people would describe them as mixed race if they walked past them on the street.

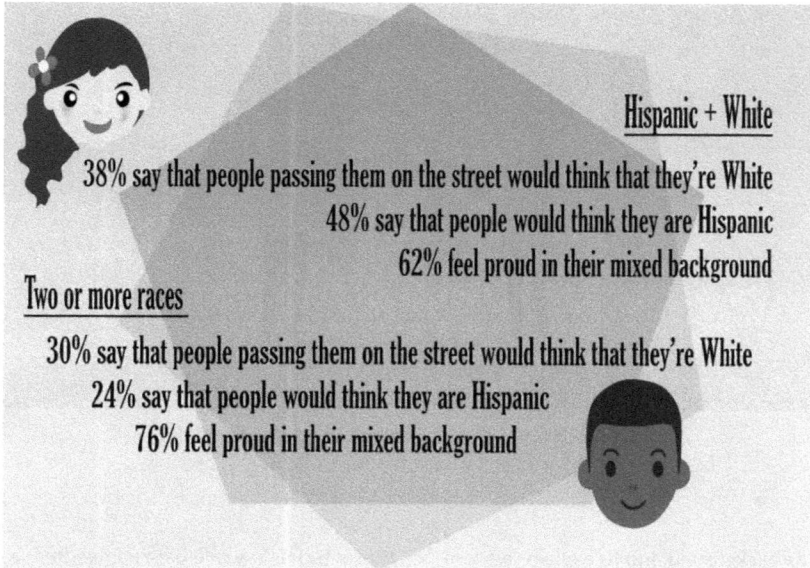

FIGURE 6. FACTORS THAT INFLUENCE HISPANIC IDENTITY: EXTERNAL PERCEPTION ACCORDING TO SELF-IDENTIFIED RACE AND ETHNICITY

Self-identified race has numerous implications. For instance, individuals who self-identify as a racial/ethnic minority but who are socially assigned as White have been reported to be more likely to receive preventive vaccination and less likely to report discrimination when they receive health care. [58]

Another group of investigators that utilized a large sample size and logistic regression to identify potential differences in self-reported health outcomes among Hispanics by asking questions such as: "How would you rate your overall physical health?" found that when one takes into account factors such as country of origin, nativity and citizenship, differences do exist particularly among Mexican Americans. More research is needed, and these studies are not without limitations, but they do raise the question of how much external perception influences the quality of healthcare among minorities. [59]

Among foreign-born Hispanics, the longer they have lived in the U.S., the less likely they are to describe themselves using the demonym for the country of origin (i.e. Mexican, Colombian, etc.). However, only 17% of Hispanics who have lived in the U.S. for 20 years or longer describe themselves as "Americans." 59% still use the demonym of the country of origin.

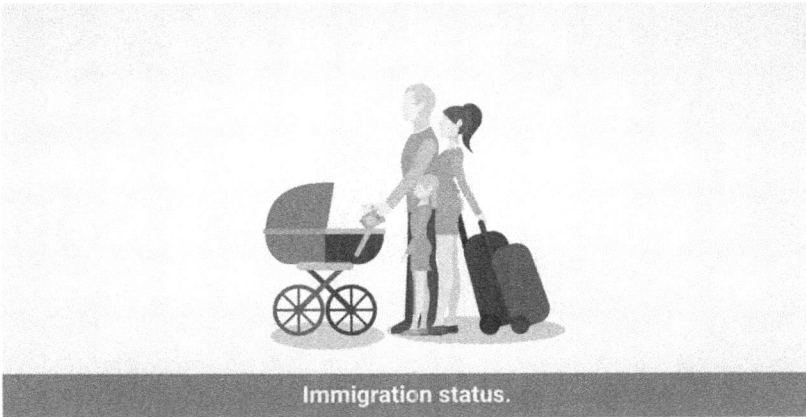

Immigration status.

FIGURE 7. FACTORS THAT INFLUENCE HISPANIC IDENTITY: IMMIGRATION STATUS

Only 8% of Hispanic immigrants say that they most often call themselves "American." That number increases to 37% in second-generation Hispanics, which is equivalent to the 38% of Hispanics who identify themselves as citizens of the country of origin.

"No particular race is the enemy. Ignorance is the enemy."
– George Lopez

The National Survey of Latinos [53] found that asking specific questions about racial background (instead of a general question about mixed race), with questions such as: "Do you consider yourself to be Afro-Latino or Afro-Hispanic (a Latino or Hispanic with Black African ancestry)?" or, "Do you consider yourself to be indigenous or Native American, (Mayan, Quechua, or some other indigenous or Native American origin)?," resulted in as many as one-third of the Latino adults saying that they consider themselves to be mixed race.

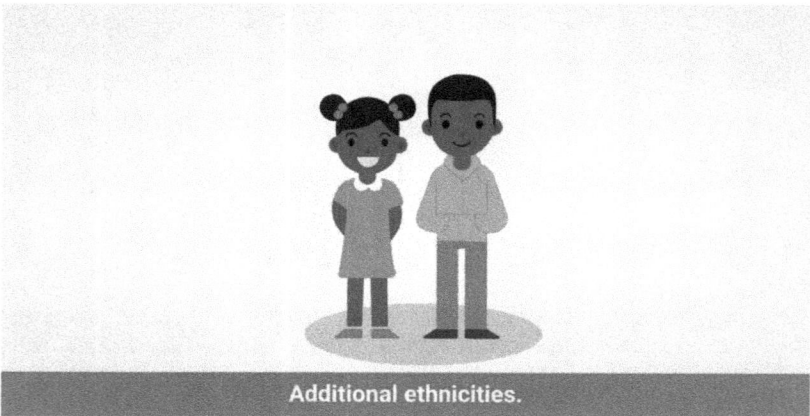

Additional ethnicities.

FIGURE 8. FACTORS THAT INFLUENCE HISPANIC IDENTITY: ADDITIONAL ETHNICITIES

About 30% of respondents in all groups said that their multiracial background has been an advantage, and more than half of the respondents said that their background has not made a difference. [57] This is an interesting finding because only 18% of non-Hispanic multiracial individuals say that their background has been an advantage, whereas 78% say it has not made a difference.

Most Hispanics surveyed by the Pew Research Center say that they "often" or "sometimes" feel proud of their mixed-race background. This is true for 76% of those who choose two or more races and 62% for those choosing one other race, compared with 58% for non-Hispanic multiracial.

Percentage of Hispanics saying that they are mixed-race

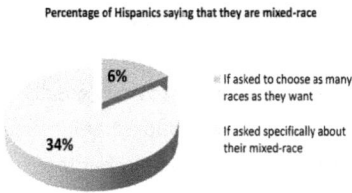

6% — If asked to choose as many races as they want

34% — If asked specifically about their mixed-race

Of note, many of these respondents indicate that one of their races is White. However, when asked to describe their race and told that they can choose as many races as the want, 6% of Hispanics say that they are "mixed race" or indicate that they are two or more races. In contrast, when specifically asked about their mixed-race, 34% say that they consider themselves to be mixed race (e.g. Mestizo, Mulatto).

Similarly, when exploring mixed-race identity using terms such as Mestizo or Mulatto, which are used in several areas of Latinoamerica to describe mixed Indigenous and European descent, 25% of 1,520 respondents consider themselves indigenous (i.e. Maya, Nahua, Taino, Quiche, Aymara, Quechua, others) and 34%

"My mother gave me one piece of advice that stuck with me. She said don't forget where you came from."
– Eva Longoria

said they are mixed-race. Importantly, it is only when asked directly about mixed-race that respondents state that they consider themselves indigenous or Native American. If the standard race question from the census is used, 41% choose White as their race or one of their races, and 30% choose Hispanic or Latino.

One aspect not often taken into account but relevant for the topic discussed here, is the fact that the broad terms *Hispanic* and *Latino* used most surveys assume that all subgroups collectively included are similar.

In reality, the variability within the Hispanic population has been proposed to be as high as the variability between Hispanics and Whites. There are differences in level of acculturation, reasons for immigrating to the U.S., socioeconomic status, racial identity perception and, as we will discuss later in this book, there are also differences in level of educational attainment and health status.

When asked whether Hispanics from different countries who live in the U.S. share similar values, the great majority said that they had either "some" or "a lot in common." But when looking at the data carefully, the responses vary greatly depending on the country of origin, the time spent in the U.S. and other factors. For example, the longer Hispanics are in the U.S., the more they believe that they have "a lot" in common with Hispanics from other countries.

Place of birth or racial identity of parents/grandparents

Considering racial identities of parents and grandparents increases the number of Hispanics identifying themselves as mixed-race even more, which again demonstrates the complexity of quantification of persons of Hispanic ethnicity. Thus, while 34% of respondents say that they are mixed-race when asked only about their own background, 40% say that they are mixed-race when their parents and grandparents are taken into consideration.

Similarly, the number of those saying that they have indigenous background goes up from 25% to 33% when the background of parents and grandparents is considered.

Even though statistical analysis was not conducted (or at least reported) in this study, and therefore I cannot claim that these differences are statistically significant, the results suggest that the racial identity of Hispanics does change when they consider their ancestors as well as themselves.

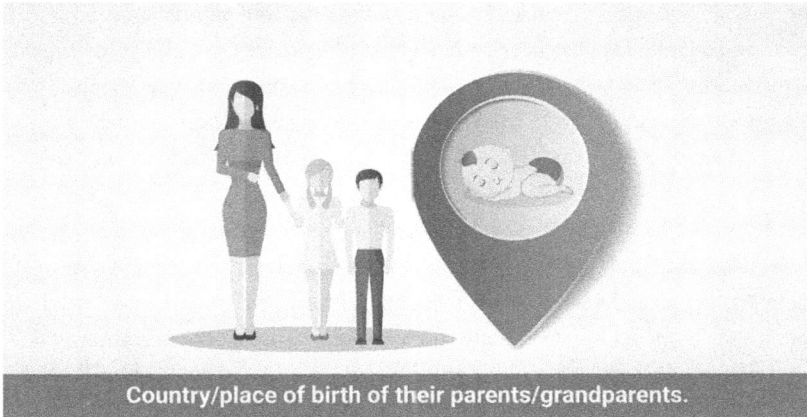

Country/place of birth of their parents/grandparents.

FIGURE 10. FACTORS THAT INFLUENCE HISPANIC IDENTITY: PLACE OF BIRTH OF FAMILY MEMBERS

Language spoken at home

40 million U.S. residents ages 5 and older speak Spanish at home. This corresponds to 13.3% of U.S. residents and represents a 133.4% increase since 1990 when the number of Spanish-speaking residents ages 5 and up was 17.3 million.

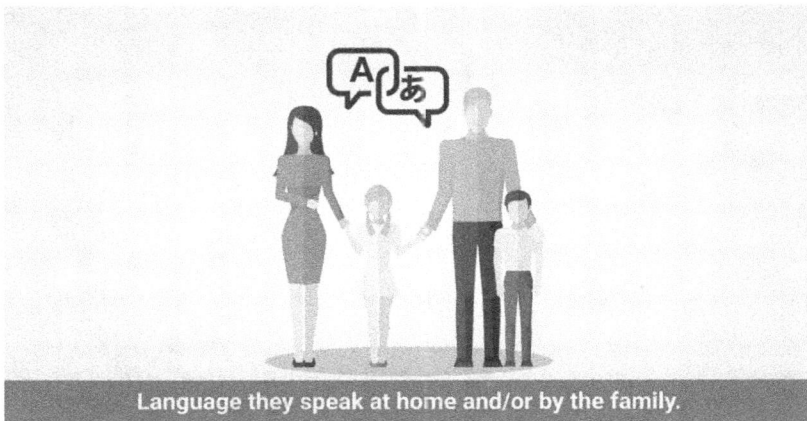

Language they speak at home and/or by the family.

FIGURE 11. FACTORS THAT INFLUENCE HISPANIC IDENTITY: LANGUAGE SPOKEN AT HOME

According to the most recent survey, **8.6% of the American population is considered limited English proficient**, meaning they speak English "less than very well." More than 23 million Spanish-speaking households report speaking English "very well" and more than 16 million report speaking English "less than very well."[29] Five percent of children ages 5 to 17 in the U.S. speak English less than "very well."

It is important to mention that even though the rates of English proficiency remain low among Hispanics overall, there have been significant changes over time. For example, the number of foreign-born Hispanic children who are English proficient has increased significantly. **Among Hispanic adults, the percentage that speaks only English at home has increased from 28% to 40% between 1980 and 2013**. [60] The potential reasons for the growth in English speakers include the increased numbers of U.S.-born Hispanics and the decrease in immigration from Latin America. Since 2000 the growth of the Hispanic population has been driven primarily by U.S. births, as opposed to new immigrants.

English proficiency in SPANISH-SPEAKING HOUSEHOLDS, selected states 2017

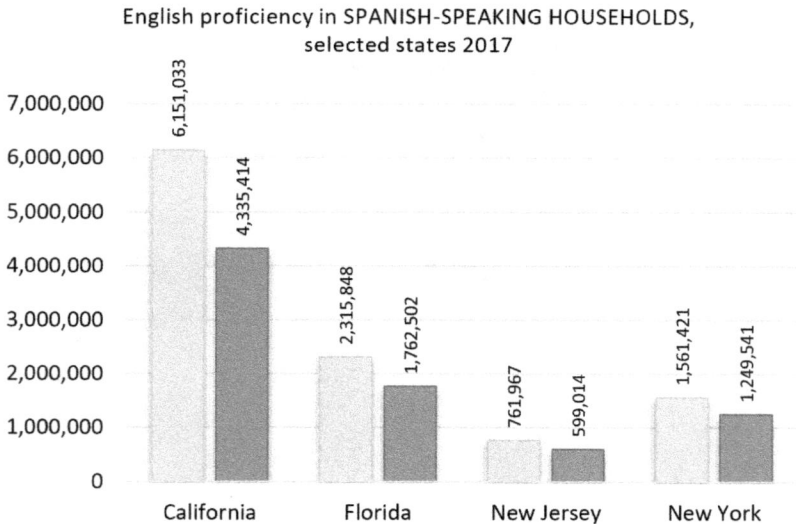

FIGURE 12. 2017 ESTIMATES OF THE NUMBER OF HOUSEHOLDS IN SELECTED STATES WHERE SPANISH IS SPOKEN. OF THOSE, THE NUMBER OF HOUSEHOLDS THAT INDICATED THAT THEY SPEAK ENGLISH "VERY WELL" OR "LESS THAN VERY WELL" IS DEPICTED. ERROR BARS ARE NOT INCLUDED. SOURCE: U.S. CENSUS BUREAU

One important consideration to the data presented in Figure 12 is that typically, information on English proficiency is not categorized by place of birth. There are clear differences between U.S. and foreign-born Hispanics in regard to language use, and failure to take those differences into consideration can result in misinterpretation of the data.

Also, even though a high percentage of foreign-born Hispanics speak Spanish at home, many also speak English "very well." As expected, a very high percentage of U.S.-born Hispanics speak English proficiently yet one-third of them speak Spanish at home. This may be related to generational and educational attainment differences among family members. According to Pew Research Center data, only 5% of foreign-born Hispanics spoke only English at home in 2013 and among Hispanics who were not proficient in English or said that they don't speak English, 52% and 75% had less than high school education, respectively. [60]

Out of the 70% of Latinos ages 5 and older who spoke English proficiently in 2017, the highest levels of English proficiency were among Spaniards (93%), Panamanians (87%) and Puerto Ricans (83%). 71% of Mexicans speak English proficiently and only approximately half of Hispanics from Central American countries such as Guatemala, El Salvador and Honduras are proficient in English. Additionally, Spanish spoken in different countries is not equal. Words have different meanings and connotations in different countries. This is relevant for interactions between physicians and their patients.

According to the 2015 survey of Latino adults conducted by the Pew Research Center, 58% of immigrant, 87% of U.S.-born, and 81% of registered voter Hispanics don't believe that speaking Spanish is a necessary component of Latino identity. [61, 62]

It is important to estimate how many Hispanics in the U.S. are not English proficient because their lack of English communication skills has a direct impact on their access to health care and their comfort with English-speaking healthcare providers. As discussed in more detail later in this book, there may be correlation between English-language proficiency and health outcomes.

Many Hispanics living in the U.S. have strong ties with their countries of origin. [21] The term "transmigrant" is used to describe immigrants who travel to their countries of origin with certain frequency, who send money to their families there, make regular phone calls there, or have children still living there.

Transmigrants who engage in these cross-border activities tend to correspond to those who do not plan to stay in the U.S. for good, consider the morals of their country to be superior to those in the U.S., and, relevant to this discussion, are less likely to describe themselves as Americans and more likely to use the demonym corresponding to their country of origin when describing their racial identity.

As expected, the longer they've lived in the U.S., the less likely it is for immigrants to behave as transmigrants. [21]

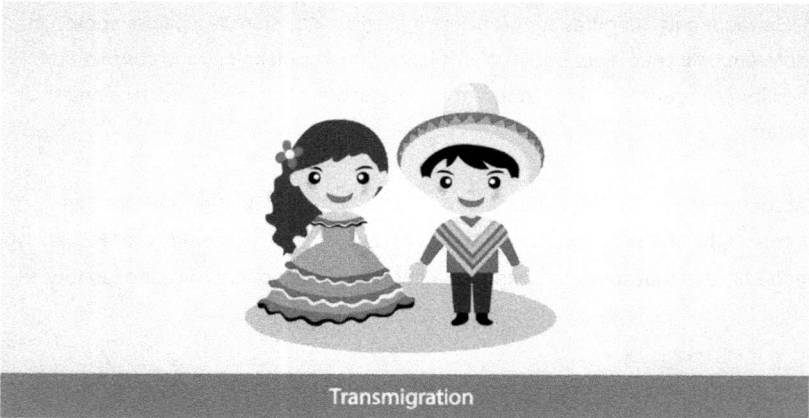
Transmigration

FIGURE 13. FACTORS THAT INFLUENCE HISPANIC IDENTITY: FAMILY TRADITIONS AND TRANSMIGRATION

Key takeaways from chapter 2

1

Most people think of "race" as a group of common inborn biological traits (e.g., skin color, shape of the face or nose, color of the eyes or hair). However, there are no biological characteristics that permit the division of each race into purely distinct categories.

2

There is a new definition of race, in which a complex combination of culture, family traditions, spoken languages, gender identity and many other factors define who we are beyond our place of birth, or that of our ancestors.

Multiple factors contribute to Hispanic identity. These include:
a. The person's generation within the U.S.: Third- and fourth-generation Hispanics are less likely to identify themselves as Hispanics.

b. External perception: Individuals who consider themselves multiracial are more likely to say that people passing them on the street would think they're Hispanic.

c. Immigration status: Individuals who have recently migrated to the U.S. are more likely to identify themselves as Hispanic and the longer they have lived in the U.S., the less likely they are to describe themselves using the demonym for the country of origin.

d. Additional ethnicities: The more time Hispanics are in the US, the more they believe that they have "a lot" in common with Hispanics from other countries.

e. Language spoken at home: Most Hispanics don't believe that speaking Spanish is a necessary component of Latino identity but it is estimated that 40 million U.S. residents ages 5 and older speak Spanish at home.

Online resources for chapter 2

IF YOU ARE INTERESTED IN:	GO TO:
National surveys with data on citizenship, literacy, heritage, etc.	The Hispanic Research Center interactive data tool: https://www.hispanicresearchcenter.org/research-resources/data-tool-unpacking-hispanic-diversity/
Public opinion polling, demographic research, media content analysis and other empirical social science research	The Pew Research Center Pew Research Center
Additional information on the past, present and future of the Spanish language in the United States, including in-depth discussions around its economic and social impact.	The Future of Spanish in the United States: The Language of Hispanic Migrant Communities by Alonso, et al.[62]
Racial-Ethnic Identity Development	EmbraceRace.org a multiracial community of parents, teachers, experts, and other caring adults who support each other to meet the challenges that race poses to our children, families, and communities.

https://www.embracerace.org/
resources/recording-and-resources-
understanding-racial-ethnic-identity-
development

The Eñye Nation Movement   https://www.enyenation.com/

https://www.enyenation.com/
resource_redirect/landing_
pages/306629

HISPANIC
EDUCATIONAL
ATTAINMENT

"Year after year, we see persistent gaps in achievement based on race and income level. These gaps do not stem from disparate ability; rather, they are the result of systems designed to perpetuate injustice."
- Elisha Smith Arrillaga, Executive Director, ED Trust West

ANA MARIA WENT TO AN ELEMENTARY SCHOOL WHERE MANY STUDENTS SPOKE SPANISH

"Spanish-speaking students went to class on the first floor. English-speaking students received more advanced classes on the second floor. Most of us spoke only Spanish at home though.

"I struggled when we first moved to the U.S., but I asked my teacher to move me to the second floor after a few months. How can you possibly improve, if they're speaking to you in Spanish not only at home but also at school?

"One of the reasons why my test scores were so low was my English deficiency, but at the time I didn't realize how much my scores would affect my chances of going to college. I was a child. All I cared about was not being made fun of by my classmates as a Spanish-speaking immigrant!"

CHAPTER THREE

THE EDUCATIONAL PIPELINE BY THE NUMBERS

How early do the disparities begin?

"The pipeline itself is just too small. The barriers exist up and down the continuum to our segregated education system.... Too many of our minority students are in poor-performing or underperforming K-12 school systems."
- Marc Nivet, chief diversity officer of the Association of American Medical Colleges (AAMC).

This chapter describes the statistics around the Hispanic representation throughout the educational pipeline in the U.S.

A few limitations must be mentioned before summarizing the data:

1. Hispanic ethnicity is defined in the census as described in chapter one and thus it may not accurately represent the Hispanic student population. In addition, different sources of data sometimes use different definitions and some definitions have been modified overtime. For example, since 2011, students participating in <u>NAEP</u> were identified by school reports as one of the seven racial/ethnic categories [63] different from the current census categorization:

- White
- Black or African American
- Hispanic
- Asian
- Native Hawaiian or Other Pacific Islander
- American Indian or Alaska Native
- Two or More Races

2. No database takes into account the multiple aspects of racial identity described in chapter two. Thus, Hispanics from all backgrounds are counted together. When available, I will describe variations for students from different backgrounds and countries of origin.

3. Disparities between White and Hispanic students have been observed since the first time the data on educational attainment started to be collected. Because the starting points were not even, looking at the so-called White-Hispanic gap at specific points in time prevents us from seeing the positive changes that have taken place, at least in some of the measures of educational attainment. I will present the longitudinal data when available, and point out changes over time using bold letters within the text.

4. Hispanic students that drop out of school early for any reason, such as economical or family reasons, are no longer included in the data at later stages of the educational journey where the disparities appear smaller.

Educational achievement and how is it defined and measured

In order to interpret the wealth of available data comparing Hispanic students with those of other races and ethnicities [63], it is as critical to understand how data on educational achievement is collected as it is to understanding how data on race and ethnicity is collected by the census. As with other topics, I will only briefly summarize key pieces of information and provide references to other more comprehensive publications on each topic for those interested. [64] A detailed description of each test is included in the Glossary.

Apart from graduation rates, which measure educational attainment at different levels, standardized testing measures achievement, that is, the progress made by a student during his or her educational journey. These tests also serve as a measure of accountability for schools, particularly low performing ones.

Standardized testing is designed, at least in theory, to ensure that all students are taught to high academic standards that will prepare them for college, taking into account equal access to instruction for disadvantaged and high-need students. For that reason, it is important to compare test scores and graduation rates between Hispanic students and students of other races and ethnicities, taking into account potential racial biases in school assessment measures.

The National Assessment of Educational Progress (NAEP) and the "White-Hispanic gap" in reading and math

The graphs below shows data on NAEP science and reading scores for White, Black and Hispanic students in 4th and 8th grade in 2015..

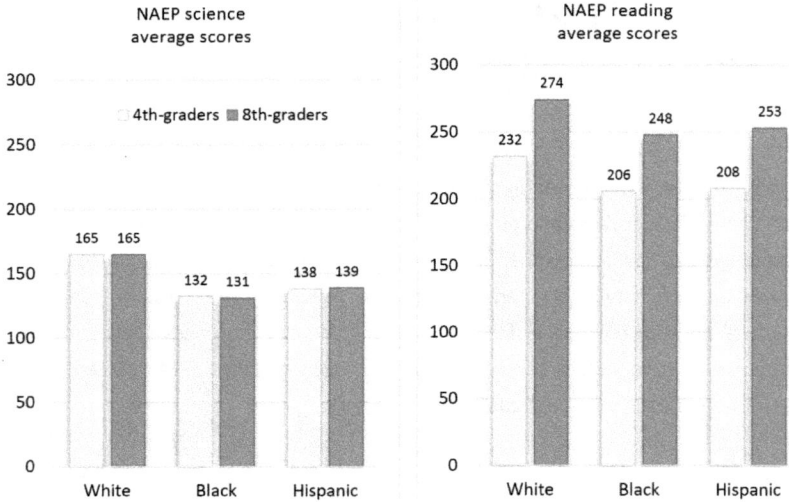

NAEP science average scores

- 4th-graders
- 8th-graders

	White	Black	Hispanic
4th-graders	165	132	138
8th-graders	165	131	139

NAEP reading average scores

	White	Black	Hispanic
4th	232	206	208
8th	274	248	253

FIGURE 14. AVERAGE NAEP SCIENCE (LEFT) AND READING (RIGHT) AVERAGE SCORES FOR 4TH (BLUE) AND 8TH (RED) GRADE BY RACE AND ETHNICITY 2015. U.S. DEPARTMENT OF EDUCATION, NATIONAL CENTER FOR EDUCATION STATISTICS, NATIONAL ASSESSMENT OF EDUCATIONAL PROGRESS (NAEP), READING ASSESSMENTS

As mentioned at the beginning of this chapter, there are caveats to the interpretation of disparities between Whites and Hispanics [63], primarily related to the fact that the data are presented at individual points in time. However, when looking at the NAEP data longitudinally, no significant changes are evident.

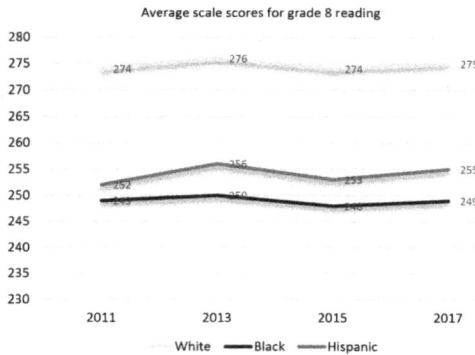

Average scale scores for grade 8 reading

FIGURE 15. AVERAGE SCALE SCORES FOR GRADE 8 READING, BY RACE/ETHNICITY USING 2011 GUIDELINES, SCHOOL-REPORTED [SRACE10] AND JURISDICTION: 2011-2017

There are two key pieces of information corresponding to the most recent dataset (2017) data are summarized below:

- The White-Hispanic gap in mathematics achievement scores (19 points) has not been measurably different since the 1990's when the NAEP was first administered.
- The White-Hispanic gap in reading at grades 4, 8 and 12, (23, 24 and 20 points, respectively) was not measurably different in 2017 compared to the gap in the 1990's.

Eighth graders who scored below proficient math achievement level by race, 2019

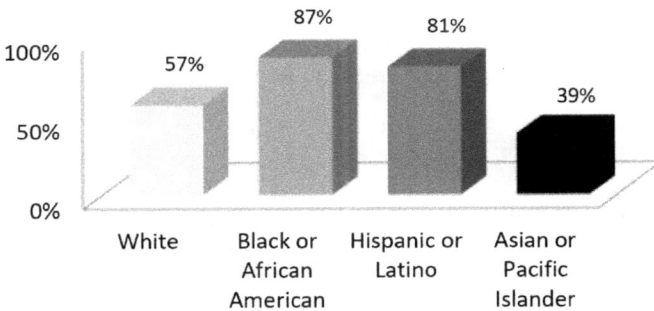

SAT, MCAT and STJs

In 2018, the average SAT scores for math were significantly lower for Hispanics compared to Whites. Even though the scores were up from the previous years for all races and ethnicities, they remained the same for Hispanics and Native Hawaiians. [65]

SAT scores, 2018

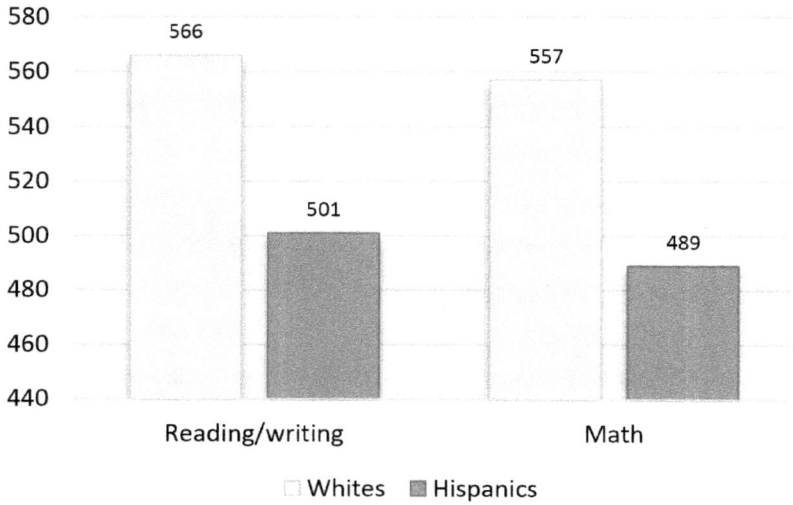

Reading/writing: Whites 566, Hispanics 501
Math: Whites 557, Hispanics 489

Whites ▢ Hispanics ▨

FIGURE 17. SAT SCORES BY RACE AND ETHNICITY, 2018

Percentage distribution of enrollment in public elementary and secondary schools, by race/ethnicity: 2010-2027

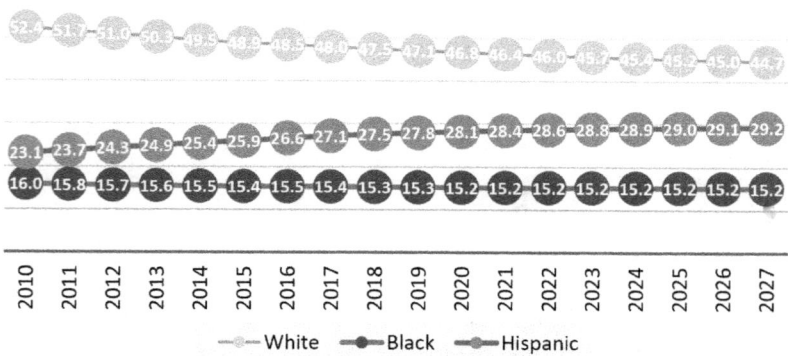

White: 52.4, 51.7, 51.0, 50.3, 49.5, 48.9, 48.5, 48.0, 47.5, 47.1, 46.8, 46.4, 46.0, 45.7, 45.4, 45.2, 45.0, 44.7

Black: 23.1, 23.7, 24.3, 24.9, 25.4, 25.9, 26.6, 27.1, 27.5, 27.8, 28.1, 28.4, 28.6, 28.8, 28.9, 29.0, 29.1, 29.2

Hispanic: 16.0, 15.8, 15.7, 15.6, 15.5, 15.4, 15.5, 15.4, 15.3, 15.3, 15.2, 15.2, 15.2, 15.2, 15.2, 15.2, 15.2, 15.2

Years: 2010, 2011, 2012, 2013, 2014, 2015, 2016, 2017, 2018, 2019, 2020, 2021, 2022, 2023, 2024, 2025, 2026, 2027

White ● Black ● Hispanic ●

FIGURE 18. SAT MEAN SCORES OF COLLEGE-BOUND SENIORS, BY RACE/ETHNICITY: SELECTED YEARS

Hispanics also score consistently lower in the MCAT than Whites. For the school year 2019-2020, the average total MCAT score for Hispanics matriculating to Medical School was 506.2, compared to 512.1 for Whites

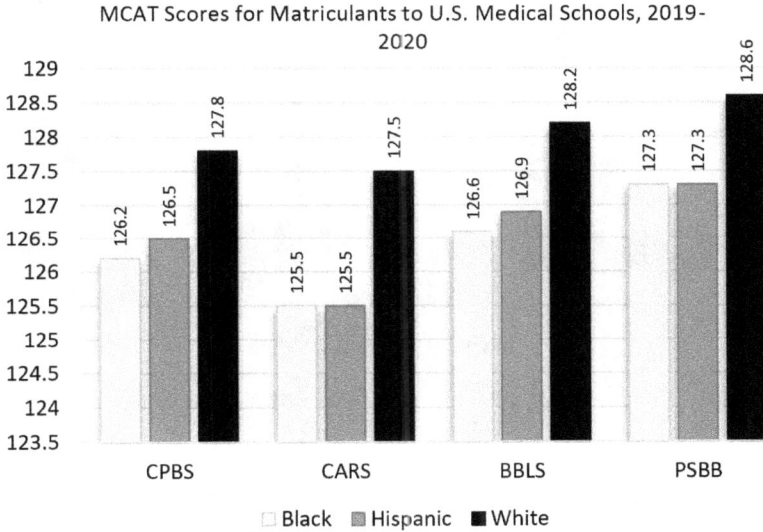

MCAT Scores for Matriculants to U.S. Medical Schools, 2019-2020

Subtest	Black	Hispanic	White
CPBS	126.2	126.5	127.8
CARS	125.5	125.5	127.5
BBLS	126.6	126.9	128.2
PSBB	127.3	127.3	128.6

FIGURE 19. MCAT SCORES AND GPAS FOR MATRICULANTS TO U.S. MEDICAL SCHOOLS BY RACE/ETHNICITY

GPA scores are lower among Hispanic students, compared to other races. In 2019-2020, the average total GPA for Hispanics matriculating to medical school was 3.62, compared to an average 3.76 for Whites.

Average GPA scores among matriculants to Medical School, 2019-2020

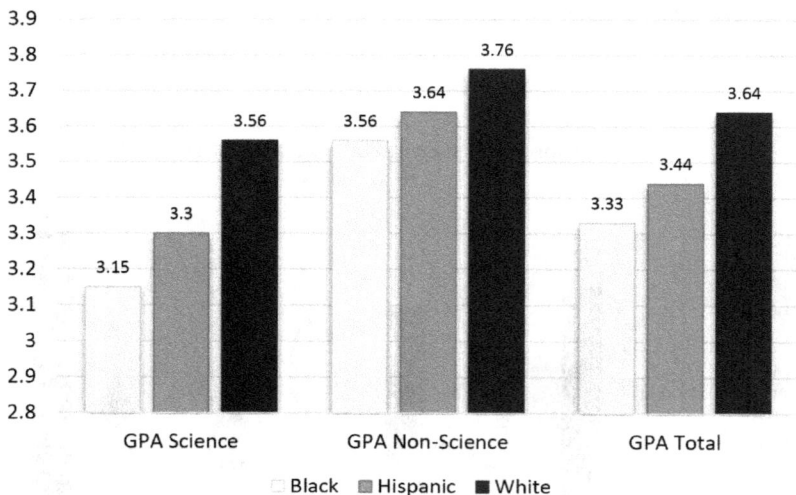

FIGURE 20. AVERAGE GPA SCORES AMONG MATRICULANTS TO MEDICAL SCHOOL, 2019-2020

Newer tests such as the California Science Test known as CAST recently conducted for the first time, showed alarmingly low scores for English learners, with only 3 percent of them meeting the standards, compared with an overall 30 percent of all students in the state who did.[66]

"We know these results are not a reflection of student ability; rather, they are a reflection of systems and practices that continue to fail students"
– Christopher J. Nellum, deputy director of Education Trust-West

Is there a racial bias in standardized testing?

A key question for our discussion is whether race and ethnicity influence scores in any way. [67] As shown above, Hispanics score lower than Whites in all tests. Because this is also the case for other minorities like Blacks, it has been stated that these tests are intrinsically biased.

I recently spoke with an undergraduate student interested in a career in medicine, who told me that all his Hispanic college friends "know" that Hispanics score lower in the SAT and the MCAT, and that admissions officials are less strict in terms of scores when reviewing applications from Hispanic students. This statement is actually in line with research around the "stereotype threat," which refers to people feeling afraid of confirming stereotypes related to their social group. For instance, it's been shown that when labeling a test as an intelligence evaluation, the scores of certain groups such as African Americans are negatively affected. These beliefs have been proposed as one of the reasons for the racial disparities, beyond a potential inherent bias associated with the test itself. [68-70]

Formal studies to determine how well the MCAT predicts long-term outcomes and whether there is a difference in its ability to predict outcomes among students of different races and ethnicities have been published. [71] suggesting that the differences seen across races is due to the inequalities throughout the students' educational journey, instead of a true racial bias that is inherent to the test. [72] As we will see in the next sections, Hispanic students are exposed to multiple risk factors for low educational attainment that contribute to their performance in standardized tests and that have nothing to do with their aptitude.

For example, it has been reported that SAT scores have strong correlations with parent's level of education and family income, putting already disadvantaged students at further disadvantage. Affluent students have access to better education, are usually native speakers and have educated parents, which gives them an advantage in the verbal part of the SAT even when controlling for socioeconomic factors, racial differences still persist. [73]

Over the years, many different approaches have been proposed to overcome potential racial or socioeconomic biases related with the SAT. From rebranding it to help decouple the test from its reputation, revising it by prioritizing certain portions of the test that appear to assess students more uniformly, replacing it by new types of testing, making test materials available for free to ensure equal access to preparatory activities, or completely eliminating the test. In fact many schools have already chosen not to use test scores in their admissions process.

In an effort to address inequalities, it was just recently announced that a new "adversity score" was going to be incorporated to the SAT. [74] This change may or may not have been related to the news related to college admissions, including the so-called "Operation Varsity Blues" scandal or the lawsuit against Harvard University for allegedly discriminating against Asian Americans during the college admissions process. The proposed "adversity score" was planned to be rolled out to 150 schools in 2020 amidst a lot of controversy around its validity. [75]

However, only a few months after this announcement, the College Board withdrew the proposal to roll-out the "adversity score," stating that they were adopting "a humbler position" and that the College Board "should keep its focus on scoring achievement." [76]

The MCAT seems to be good at predicting grades and USMLE outcomes. According to a recent survey, while 60% or more of all participants don't believe that race and ethnicity should be factors in college admissions decisions, the majority (67%) do believe that high school grades and test scores (47%) should be major factors.[77] Some students with lower GPAs perform well in the MCAT and some schools use MCAT scores to decide who needs more help to succeed in medical school, not to predict who will succeed in medical school. [78]

Apart from all the issues described here, one could ask whether a single test score could possibly be sufficient to predict how well suited a student is to become a doctor. The range of MCAT scores that is associated with success is wide. What this means is that you may score on the lower end of the range and do as well in medical school as someone scoring on the high end of that range. This is why schools should consider characteristics other than test scores exclusively. [79]

"We've got to admit the truth that wealth inequality has progressed to such a degree that it isn't fair to look at test scores alone. You must look at them in context of the adversity students' face."

– David Coleman, Chief Executive of the College Board

New types of tests such as the Situational Judgment Tests (SJT), which measure an individual's reactions to specific situations that they could encounter in their actual job, have been shown to be reliable and valid and they seem to provide an added value especially when used in combination with knowledge tests. [80, 81]

Until there's an assessment or group of assessments that have been validated to demonstrate their ability to predict long-term outcomes, it is clear that these tests are often used beyond their intent. I believe that colleges do well to take into account all aspects of a students' profile, including more than one measure of high school achievement as well as extra-curricular activities that support their development as more well-rounded individuals by exposing them to the world in a way that school cannot.

As we will see in the next few sections, in spite of the so-called White-Hispanic gap and the disparities in test scores described so far, there has been significant improvement in academic attainment among Hispanics over the years. I will present the overall data on educational attainment over time, by race and ethnicity, followed by key pieces of information on each step in the educational journey from elementary school through high school and college. The chapter ends with data on medical school and clinical practice, including a discussion on how sufficiency in the physician workforce is calculated.

Standardized testing and English proficiency

Students with limited-English proficiency score lower in standardized tests in reading and math at all grade levels. [82] Students with low English proficiency start behind, making it less likely that they'll be eligible for advanced classes. This topic is related to the research around the distinction between disability and difference. Many children incorrectly labeled as having a learning disability, simply need to be taught differently, addressing factors such as the language barrier. [83, 84] This is important because some researchers have shown that Hispanic children underperform African Americans at the earliest stages of academic assessment, but this is likely due to the fact that these kindergarteners are tested in English at a point in time when they do not yet speak the language. This is not only true for immigrant students, but also for children who live in households where Spanish is the primary language and are not accustomed to reading or writing in English. Children with lower reading ability at this stage are likely to be placed in lower reading groups in the first grade where they cover less material than their peers in high level reading groups, and in some cases their entry into kindergarten is delayed until they can pass screening tests. Both approaches affect their entire educational trajectory putting them at an even larger disadvantage. [85]

Educational attainment among Hispanics

Educational attainment refers to the highest level of education completed by an individual or group e.g. a college degree. This statistic is important because it is related to indicators of progress such as employment and household income.

Hispanics, more often than Whites, say that obtaining a college degree is necessary to get ahead in life (86% versus 69%). [86] Yet, according to data from the ACS, most Hispanics (6 out of 10) achieved a high school diploma or lower in 2017. [87]

Among Hispanics who have high school education or less and are not enrolled in school, 74% say that the reason they are not continuing their education is that they need to help support their family; 40% say that they cannot afford to go to school, and 49% say that their English fluency is low.

Hispanics are below all other races in educational attainment as shown in **Figure 21**. By 2017, Hispanic and Black young adults were half as likely to have completed a bachelor's degree as non-Hispanic Whites.

However, between 2000 and 2017 **the number of Hispanic students who had completed high school or higher increased** from 63% to about 83%, **the number of students who achieved an Associate's or higher degree increased** from 16% to 27.7% and **the number of Hispanics achieving a Bachelor's degree or higher increased** from 9.5% to 18.5%. The most recent data on educational attainment released on March 30, 2020 shows that 18.8% of Hispanics age 25 and older had a bachelor's degree or higher, up from 13.9% in 2010. Furthermore, it's been reported that **the number of Hispanic students enrolled in schools, colleges and universities in the United States doubled in 20 years** from 8.8 million to 17.9 million between 1996 and 2016.

Changes in educational attainment overtime, by race/ethnicity 2006-2017

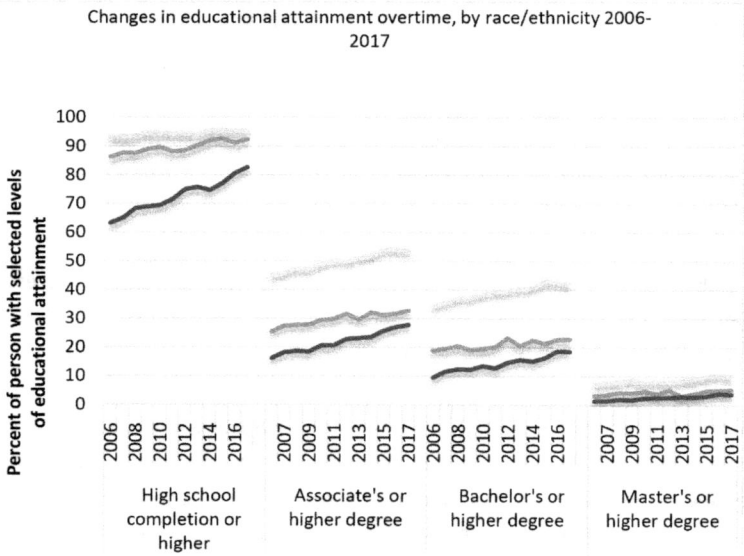

FIGURE 21. PERCENTAGE OF PERSONS 25 TO 29 YEARS OLD WITH SELECTED LEVELS OF EDUCATIONAL ATTAINMENT, BY RACE/ ETHNICITY AND SEX: SELECTED YEARS SOURCE: U.S. DEPARTMENT OF COMMERCE, CENSUS BUREAU, U.S. CENSUS OF POPULATION; CURRENT POPULATION REPORTS, VARIOUS YEARS; AND CURRENT POPULATION SURVEY (CPS)

Most metrics demonstrate that the highest unmet need is among English language learners and economically disadvantaged students. The Adjusted Cohort Graduation Rate ACGR is a newer measure of educational attainment. The 2016–17 ACGR for all students was 84.6%. The rates by subgroup are as follows:

1. 88.6% for White students,
2. 80.0% for Hispanic students,
3. 77.8% for Black students,
4. 78.3% for economically disadvantaged students,
5. 66.4% for limited English proficiency students.

In 2019, children from racial and ethnic minority groups were projected to make up 52.9% of public K-12 students, up from 35.2% in the 1990's. In fact, the number of K-12 public school minority students (i.e., Hispanic, Black and Asian Americans) has been higher than the White student population since 2014. Approximately 28% of all students enrolled in K-12 public schools were Hispanic in 2019, up from 14% in 1995. [88]

In 2017, the percentage of Hispanic students enrolled in kindergarten was 20%. This number is projected to increase further according to the 2027 projections of the National Center for Education Statistics. [88]

There is significant variability when comparing private schools with schools with high racial/ethnic concentration in which Hispanics account for 10% and 60% of all students, respectively. [87]

Percentage distribution of enrollment in public elementary and secondary schools, by race/ethnicity: 2010-2027

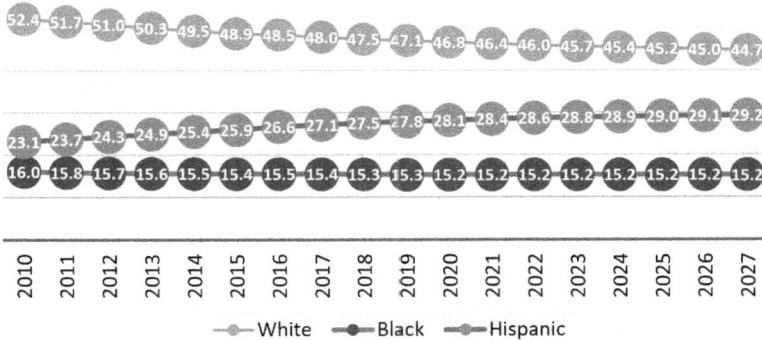

White: 52.4, 51.7, 51.0, 50.3, 49.5, 48.9, 48.5, 48.0, 47.5, 47.1, 46.8, 46.4, 46.0, 45.7, 45.4, 45.2, 45.0, 44.7

Hispanic: 23.1, 23.7, 24.3, 24.9, 25.4, 25.9, 26.6, 27.1, 27.5, 27.8, 28.1, 28.4, 28.6, 28.8, 28.9, 29.0, 29.1, 29.2

Black: 16.0, 15.8, 15.7, 15.6, 15.5, 15.4, 15.5, 15.4, 15.3, 15.3, 15.2, 15.2, 15.2, 15.2, 15.2, 15.2, 15.2, 15.2

2010, 2011, 2012, 2013, 2014, 2015, 2016, 2017, 2018, 2019, 2020, 2021, 2022, 2023, 2024, 2025, 2026, 2027

White — Black — Hispanic

FIGURE 22. PERCENTAGE DISTRIBUTION OF ENROLLMENT IN PUBLIC AND ELEMENTARY AND SECONDARY SCHOOLS SOURCE: U.S. DEPARTMENT OF EDUCATION, NATIONAL CENTER FOR EDUCATION STATISTICS, PRIVATE SCHOOL. UNIVERSE SURVEY (PSS), 2015–16. SEE DIGEST OF EDUCATION STATISTICS 2017

High school interventions have been a major focus when trying to address racial and ethnic disparities. However, research has suggested that intervening in High school may be too late. This is because dropouts begin in middle school and students from elementary schools that do not offer high-level classes, and students who start behind due to poor reading skills or language barriers, have trouble catching up later on. [89]

Evidently, academic achievement is not the only reason for students to dropout. Among minority students, the need to help support their families is an important factor. Not surprisingly, it's been shown that students who work 20 hours or more per week tend to have lower grades and to drop out more frequently. [90]

Four things to know with regard to Hispanics and high school:

1. The percentage of adults age 25 and over who had not completed high school was higher for Hispanic adults (33%) than for adults in any other racial/ethnic group in 2016.

2. Although the Hispanic completion rate remained lower than the White rate (89% versus 94%), the White-Hispanic gap narrowed between 2000 and 2016. In fact, **Hispanics experienced the greatest growth in high school status completion rate, increasing from 61.9% in 1996 to 89.1% in 2016, and the public high school graduation rate for Hispanic students increased from 75.2% to 79.3% between 2013 and 2016.**

3. When comparing all races and ethnicities, **the largest increase in total number of public high school graduates has taken place among Hispanic students.** Between 2000 and 2012 that growth was higher than 110% and according to the projections, this group will experience around 30% additional growth by 2025, which means that Hispanics will represent almost a quarter of all public high school graduates by 2025–26.

4. Even though the **Hispanic status dropout rate** among 16- to 24-year-olds has remained higher than the Black and White rates, it **has decreased among Hispanics from 28% to 9% since the early 2000's**. However, it is important to clarify that the rate is not uniform across Hispanic subgroups. For example, Peruvian descent students had the lowest dropout rate in 2016 at 2.4%, while Guatemalan descent students had the highest rate at 22.9%. [87]

College

More Hispanics are going to college, and their graduation rates are rising.

Six things to know about Hispanics and college:

1. **Hispanic young adults experienced the largest increase in college enrollment from 20.1% in 1996 to 36% in 2017**. As with the high school data, there are differences in enrollment rates among Hispanics of different backgrounds. Those of South American background enrolled at the highest rates (close to 60%), while those of Salvadorian and Puerto Rican background enrolled at the lowest rates (30.4 and 33.4, respectively). **Between 2000 and 2017, Hispanic undergraduate enrollment more than doubled** (a 142% increase from 1.4 million to 3.3 million students). In contrast, even though the enrollment for most other racial/ethnic groups increased during the first part of this period, it decreased around 2010. For example, compared with 71% in 2000, only 57% of college students were White in 2016.

2. **Among Hispanics, each 10-year age cohort had higher rates of college attainment than the next-oldest group**. Thus, the percentage of Hispanic adults with a college degree in 2017 is as follows:

* 25- to 34-year-olds 28.0%

"Institutions of higher education have an obligation, first and foremost to create the best possible educational environment for the young adults whose lives are likely to be significantly changed during their years."
— Patricia Gurin (91)

- 35- to 44-year-olds 25.8%
- 45- to 54-year-olds 25.1%
- 55- to 64-year-olds 23.5%
- 65 and older 19.5%.

3. **The number of bachelor's degrees awarded to Hispanic students more than tripled between 2000–01 and 2015–16.**

4. **Hispanic undergraduates are among the most likely to pursue and complete an associate degree**. The representation of Hispanic students increased from 10.3% of all undergraduates in the mid-1990s to 19.8% in 2016, which corresponds to the largest increase of any racial or ethnic group.

High School and College

Percentage of persons 25 to 29 years old with selected levels of educational attainment, by race/ Ethnicity and sex: 2017

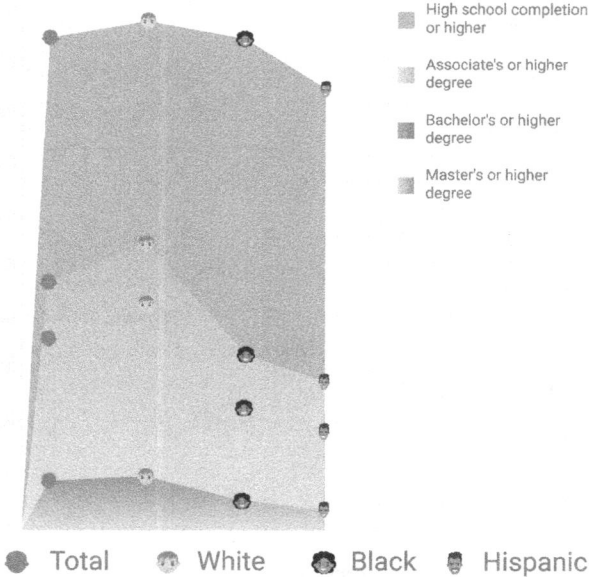

High school completion or higher

Associate's or higher degree

Bachelor's or higher degree

Master's or higher degree

Total   White   Black   Hispanic

SOURCE: Current Population Survey (CPS), Annual Social and Economic Supplement

FIGURE 23. PERCENTAGE OF PERSONS 25-29 YEARS OLD WITH SELECTED LEVELS OF EDUCATIONAL ATTAINMENT BY RACE/ ETHNICITY, 2017

One important question when looking at the trajectories of school progression is how many students who graduate high school go on to enroll into college. **In 2016, Hispanic recent high school or equivalent graduates experienced the largest increase in college enrollment among all races from 57.6% in 1996 to 70.6%**.

Hispanics are the least likely to complete their degree in health care fields.

This is great news, and in line with the observation so far that educational attainment among Hispanics is improving significantly. However, relevant to this book, this is not true for all fields of study.

Bachelor's degrees in health professions conferred by postsecondary institutions, by race/ethnicity 2016-17

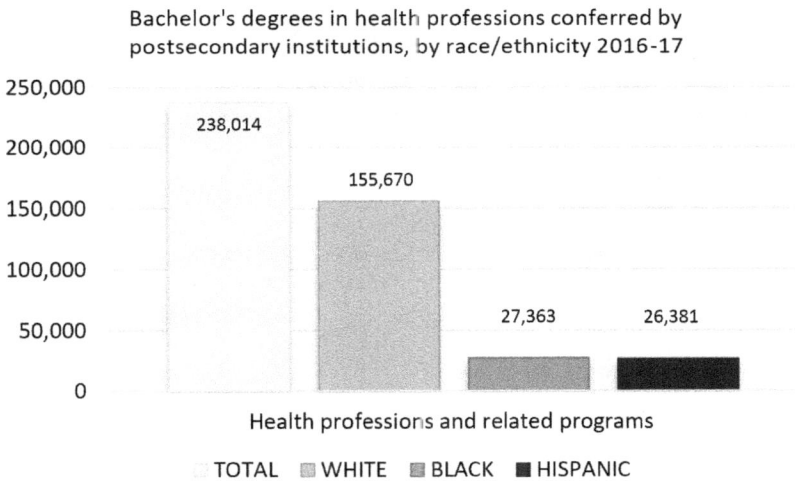

FIGURE 24. PERCENTAGE OF BACHELOR'S DEGREES CONFERRED IN SCIENCE, TECHNOLOGY, ENGINEERING, AND MATHEMATICS (STEM) FIELDS BY RACE AND ETHNICITY, 2016-2017

As shown in **Figure 24**, 65% of all bachelor's degrees in health professions were earned by Whites, compared with 11% for Blacks and Hispanics.

When looking at Post-baccalaureate degree programs which include master's and doctoral programs, as well as programs such as law, medicine, and dentistry, between 2000 and 2017, **Hispanic enrollment more than doubled from 111,000 to 275,000 students or a 148% increase**. The distribution of enrollment as a percentage of total enrollments increased from 6% to 10% among Hispanics. The on-time graduation rates in the 2016–17 school year were: 91% among Asians, 89% among non-Hispanic whites; 80% among Hispanics and 78% among non-Hispanic black students.

One interesting study looked at 15,000 students matriculating to California colleges in 1999 and 2000. [92] 11.6% of the matriculants were Hispanics. What the study found was that Latino students received significantly lower grades on average in premedical gateway courses than white students. However, they seemed to be less deterred than white students by receiving low grades in their gateway classes. After accounting for the lower grades in their initial courses, these students were more likely than white students to complete four or more gateway courses. In the words of the investigators: **"Many URM students at the campuses studied did not seem to simply give up on their career aspirations and abandon a pre-health curriculum in the face of academic adversity."**

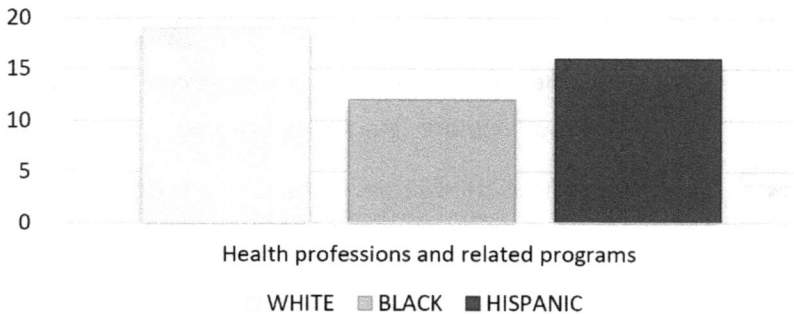

Percentage of bachelor's degrees conferred in science, technology, engineering, and mathematics (STEM) fields: 2016–17

Health professions and related programs

WHITE   BLACK   HISPANIC

FIGURE 25. PERCENTAGE OF BACHELOR'S DEGREES CONFERRED IN SCIENCE, TECHNOLOGY, ENGINEERING, AND MATHEMATICS (STEM) FIELDS BY RACE AND ETHNICITY, 2016-2017

When looking at data on bachelor's degrees conferred in all STEM fields, which include biological and biomedical sciences, computer and information sciences, engineering and engineering technologies, mathematics and statistics, and physical sciences and science technologies, the highest percentages correspond to Asians (34%) and non-resident aliens (30%), but the numbers are not as different among other races and ethnicities i.e., 19% for Whites, 16% for Hispanics and 12% for Blacks (Figure 25) as they are in health care fields.

It is estimated that by 2018, 2.4 million STEM jobs would go unfilled. With STEM jobs paying higher than other jobs, this represents a dramatic loss of opportunity.

Medical school

The main function of medical schools is to educate physicians to care for the national population. This goal can only be met if:

1. A sufficient number of physicians graduate to meet the needs of a growing population,
2. Physicians are geographically distributed in a way that the population can access care, regardless of their location,
3. Racial and ethnic minorities are represented sufficiently to meet the needs for culturally and linguistically competent care.

In the next paragraphs, I will examine each of these conditions first by describing the current demographics of medical school applicants, matriculants and graduates, followed by a discussion on geographical distribution of existing health care providers which is a factor that affects the sufficiency of the health care workforce differently in different parts of the country. The topic of culturally competent care will be addressed in Section 3.

In 2019-2020, out of 53,371 total applicants to medical school, **5,858 were Hispanics**. Of those, 2,530 students (**43.1%**) were accepted. In comparison, during the same period, **27,795 whites applied** and 12,486 (**44.92%**) students were accepted. The number of matriculants mirrors the number of applicants. Thus, 47% of matriculants in 2019-2020 were White, 7% were Black, and 6% were Hispanics.

As shown in Figure 26, the number of applicants varies significantly by country of origin mirroring the corresponding U.S. population from each country. That is, Mexicans, Puerto Ricans and Cubans are the top three countries of origin for the Hispanic population in the U.S.

HISPANIC MEDICAL SCHOOL APPLICANTS BY COUNTRY, 2015

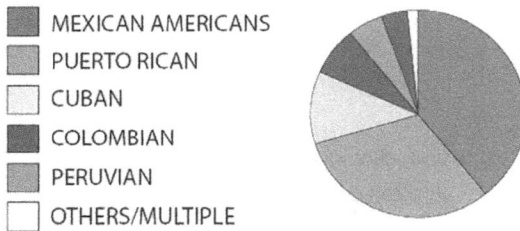

MEXICAN AMERICANS
PUERTO RICAN
CUBAN
COLOMBIAN
PERUVIAN
OTHERS/MULTIPLE

FIGURE 26. HISPANIC MEDICAL SCHOOL APPLICANTS BY COUNTRY OF ORIGIN

In order to determine the parity between the number of young adults (college age) and the number of medical school applicants and matriculants, we need to go back to 2017 for available census estimates from the ACS.

In 2017 the U.S. population of 18- to 24-year-olds was 54% (16,499,000) White and 22% (6,728,000) Hispanic. Meanwhile, out of 21,326 medical school matriculants in the same year, 49.6% (10,582) were White, while 6.4% (1,383) were Hispanic, and 7.05% (1,504) were Black.

The diversity of the young adult population does not match the diversity of medical school matriculants

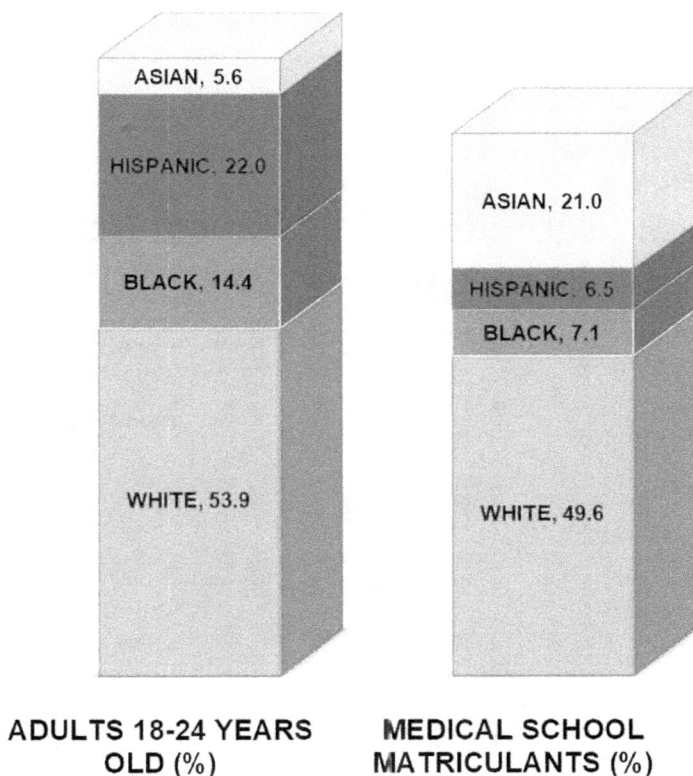

ADULTS 18-24 YEARS OLD (%)

- ASIAN, 5.6
- HISPANIC, 22.0
- BLACK, 14.4
- WHITE, 53.9

MEDICAL SCHOOL MATRICULANTS (%)

- ASIAN, 21.0
- HISPANIC, 6.5
- BLACK, 7.1
- WHITE, 49.6

FIGURE 27. U.S. YOUNG ADULT POPULATION VERSUS MEDICAL SCHOOL MATRICULANTS, BY RACE AND ETHNICITY, 2017

The acceptance rate that year was 42.5% for Hispanics and 46.1% for Whites and thus, the difference between the two is not related to differences in the number of students accepted to medical school.

While Hispanics represent 22% of the young adult population of the U.S., they only represent 6% of the medical school matriculants. In contrast, Whites represent 53.9% of the young adult population and 49.6% of the medical school matriculants. Asians represent only 5.6% of the young adult population, and 21% of the medical school matriculants

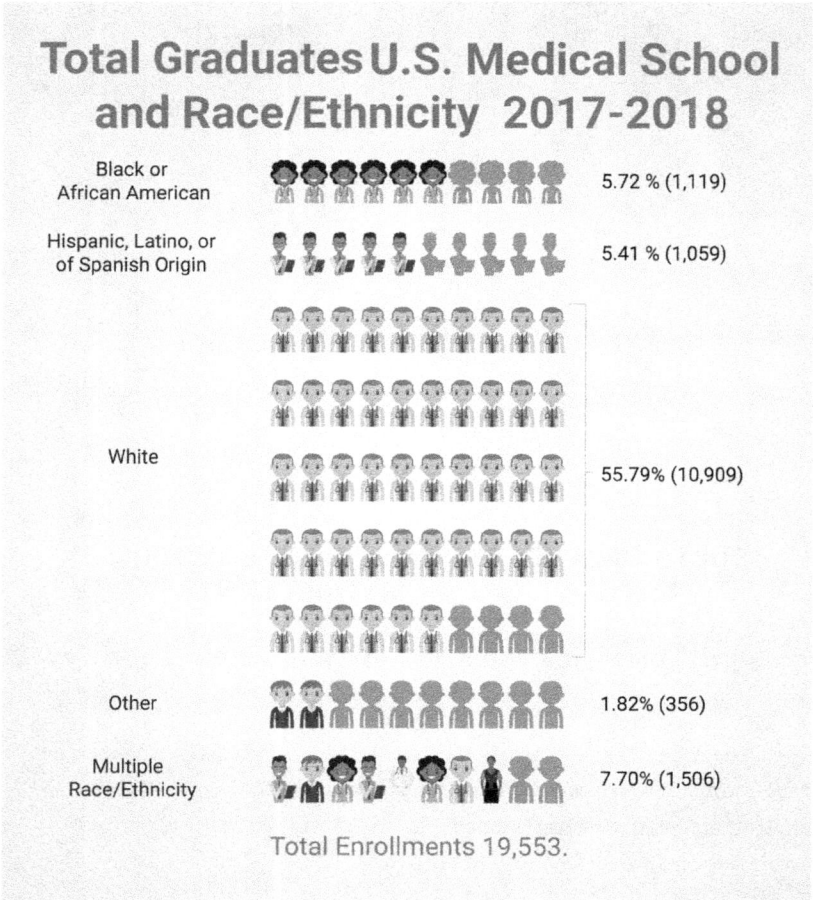

Total Graduates U.S. Medical School and Race/Ethnicity 2017-2018

Black or African American	5.72 % (1,119)
Hispanic, Latino, or of Spanish Origin	5.41 % (1,059)
White	55.79% (10,909)
Other	1.82% (356)
Multiple Race/Ethnicity	7.70% (1,506)

Total Enrollments 19,553.

FIGURE 28. TOTAL GRADUATES IN U.S. MEDICAL SCHOOLS BY RACE AND ETHNICITY 2017-2018. THE GRAPH DOES NOT INCLUDE ALL RACES FOR SIMPLICITY

RESIDENCY

Residency Applicants from U.S. MD-Granting Medical Schools to
ACGME-Accredited Programs by Specialty and Race/Ethnicity, 2018-2019

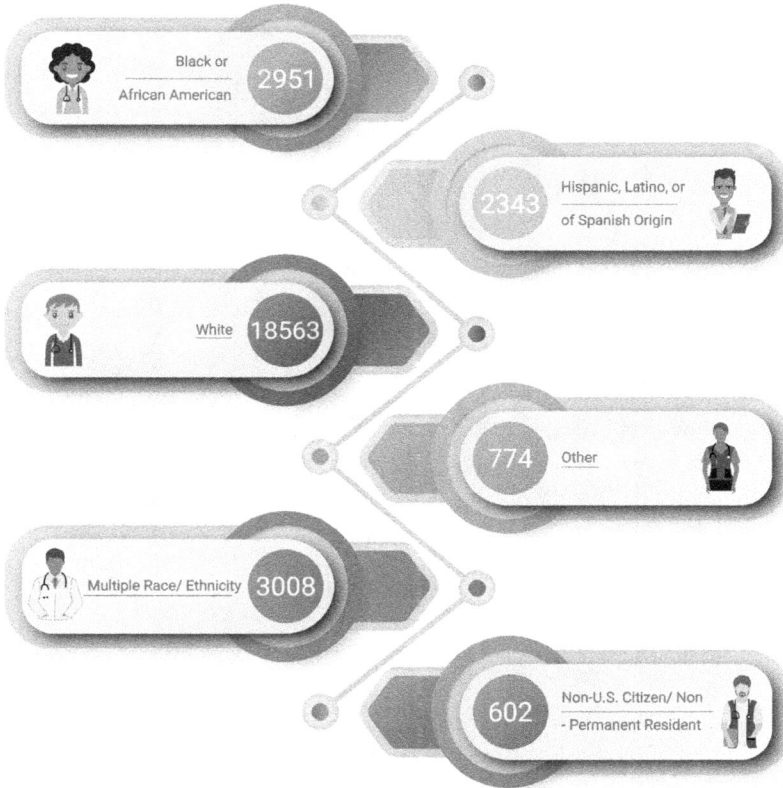

Black or African American **2951**

2343 Hispanic, Latino, or of Spanish Origin

White **18563**

774 Other

Multiple Race/ Ethnicity **3008**

602 Non-U.S. Citizen/ Non - Permanent Resident

FIGURE 29. RESIDENCY APPLICANTS FROM U.S. MD-GRANTING MEDICAL SCHOOLS TO ACGME-ACCREDITED PROGRAMS BY SELECTED SPECIALTY AND RACE/ETHNICITY. THE GRAPH SHOWS % OF TOTAL APPLICANTS PER SPECIALTY THE GRAPH DOES NOT INCLUDE ALL RACES FOR SIMPLICITY. CREATED USING DATA FROM THE AAMC

The Electronic Residency Application Service (ERS), which is a centralized service to apply to residencies and fellowships, has collected self-reported race and ethnicity data since the 2013-2014 academic year. In figure 30, depicting the percent of applicants by race and ethnicity across specialties that physicians most often apply to, the numbers for Hispanics are shown in red.

Residency Applicants from U.S. MD-Granting Medical Schools to ACGME-Accredited Programs by selected Specialty and Race/Ethnicity (percent of total)

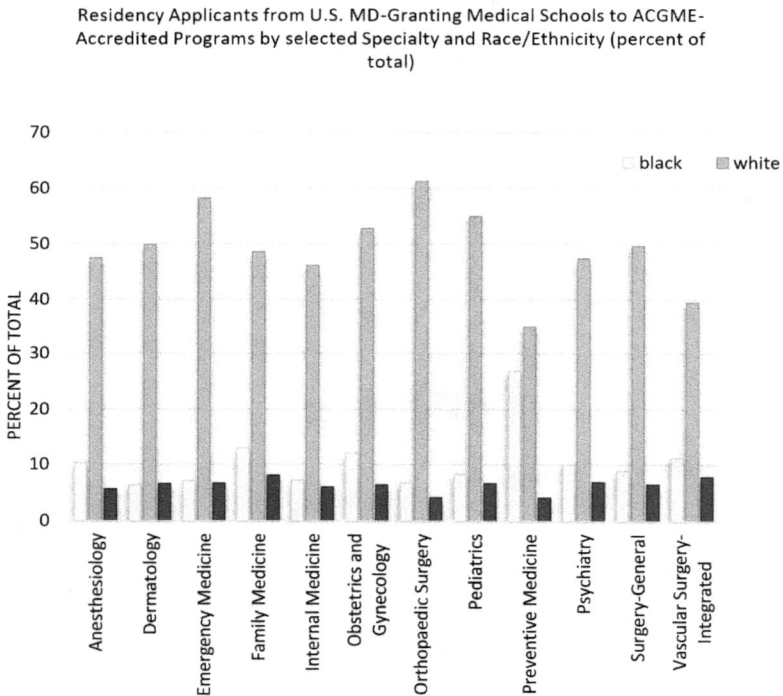

FIGURE 30. RESIDENCY APPLICANTS FROM U.S. MD-GRANTING MEDICAL SCHOOLS BY SPECIALTY AND RACE/ETHNICITY 2018-2019

A recent diversity and inclusion exercise [93] conducted by the Accreditation Council for Graduate Medical Education (ACGME) and the Council of Review Committee residents (CRCR) composed of residents from each medical specialty, revealed several issues that their membership considers may affect physicians in training, including:

1. Microaggressions: members stating that they were mistaken as cleaning staff or being complimented for speaking "good English."
2. Inadequacy of cultural competence training.
3. Underreporting of workplace discrimination for fear of retaliation.
4. Tolerance of inadequate behaviors due to the seniority of the aggressor at their institution.

Similar findings have been reported from surveys conducted among faculty and medical school leaders. [94]

Physicians in clinical practice and faculty positions

If the determination of the size of the Hispanic population is challenging as described in Section One of this book, accurately determining how many healthcare providers are needed in the short- and longer-term is even more difficult. I will start this section by discussing how the sufficiency of the workforce is estimated, to explain why we say that there is a shortage of Hispanic physicians in the U.S.

In the United States, the Health Resources and Service Administration's (HRSA) is the organization devoted to improving health and achieving health equity. One of its key objectives is to strengthen the health workforce to meet the needs of an increasingly diverse U.S. population.

The HRSA publishes a brief document on the distribution of sex and race/ethnicity in health occupations in the U.S. Here are some definitions used in their analyses:
1. The U.S. workforce is defined as those who are 16 years or older, and are currently employed or seeking employment.
2. Diversity in health occupations is measured by the representation of minority groups in a health occupation relative to their representation in the U.S. workforce.

3.   Health occupations are divided in 6 categories. Physicians are part of the
     "Health Diagnosing and Treating Practitioners" category.

In their most recent brief published in 2017 corresponding to ACS data obtained
between 2011 and 2015, the HRSA reports that Whites make up the majority of
the U.S. workforce (64.4%) compared to Hispanics (16.1%), and Blacks or African
Americans (11.6%).

**The 2017 ACS shows that 67% of the physicians in the workforce were White, and
6.3% Hispanic.**

Using data corresponding to the percentage of active physicians as of July 1st, 2019,
the AAMC reports that 5.8% of physicians were Hispanic, 56.2% White, 5% Black or
African American, and 17.1% Asian.

Distribution of Physicians by Race/Ethnicity relative to the working
age population (source: HRSA ACS PUMS 2011-2015)

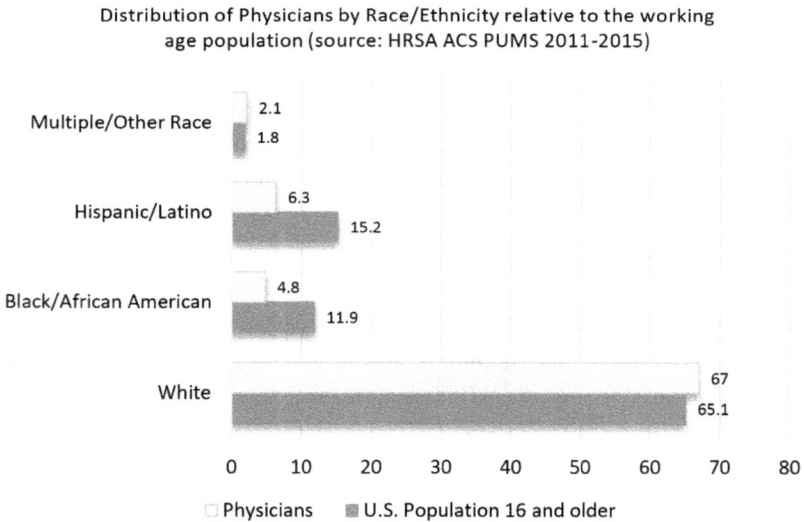

FIGURE 31. DISTRIBUTION OF PHYSICIANS BY RACE/ETHNICITY RELATIVE TO THE WORKING AGE POPULATION (SOURCE: HRSA ACS
PUMS 2011-2015)

The report concludes: *"Hispanics are significantly underrepresented in Health Diagnosing and Treating Practitioners occupations."* Within the medical professions, Public Health is the only field where the proportion of underrepresented minorities approaches population parity.

Physicians in full-time faculty positions are also mostly White (63.9%) and Asian (19.2%). Only 5.5% are Hispanic and 3.6% Black. This is true for physicians in academic appointments at all levels of academic medicine, with Hispanics representing less than 3% of all chairpersons, professors and deans, compared to more than 80% for Whites. [95] Nevertheless, it has been reported that less than a third of medical schools have programs targeting underrepresented minority faculty to enhance recruitment, promotion and retention and to provide opportunities for mentorship. [96-108]

In essence, the nation has experienced a significant demographic shift towards increased racial and ethnic diversity, while the physician workforce has not kept pace.

How is the sufficiency of the healthcare workforce determined?

There is no gold standard for assessing the sufficiency of the healthcare workforce and there's limited data on relevant supply and demand drivers specific to Hispanics, other than the projected increase in the size of the population. For example, little is known about Hispanics' current health service utilization by age and sex. Additionally, little is known about how health care needs have changed within this group over time. However, in this section I will attempt to describe some of the methods typically used to assess gaps between the supply and demand of health care providers and summarize their findings to determine whether the data supports the idea that there is a shortage of Hispanic physicians in the U.S.

Workforce planning does not appropriately measure, and likely underestimates, Hispanic healthcare provider shortages. However, **by all existing measures there is a shortage of Hispanic physicians in the U.S.**

In today's world, big data and **healthcare predictive analytics** are being used to fairly accurately predict individual aspects of the health care supply and demand continuum. For instance, it is possible to predict the number of patient visits that a hospital may receive for the next couple of months. However, these technologies have not been broadly used for workforce sufficiency, or to examine the long-term needs within specific racial/ethnic populations such as Hispanics.

Worker Density

Healthcare worker density is a measure defined by the World Health organization (WHO) as the number of health workers per 1,000 population (often reported in the literature as number per 10,000 or 100,000), and is one of the key 100 core health indicators established by the WHO. [109]

Using U.S. census data, Sanchez, G, et al, reported that **in 2010 there were 10.5 Hispanic physicians per 10,000 population in the U.S. compared to 31.5 per 10,000 non-Hispanic Whites**. [110] Furthermore, they showed that the number had declined to 10.5 from 13.5/10,000 in 1980, a 22% decline compared with a 45% increase in non-Hispanic white physicians during the same time period.*

*numbers from publication converted to n/10,000 to facilitate comparisons with other published rates

Determination of future demand is even more complex. [111, 112] In the absence of a precise tool for long-term workforce planning, estimations of the number of physicians needed 30 or 50 years down the road are unlikely to be reliable, as they are based on assumptions regarding events in the future that are difficult to predict with certainty. For example, as we'll see in the next section, calculations of workforce sufficiency and workforce planning exercises are often based on demographic evolution, i.e. the country's rate of population growth, along with the current number of physicians.

A country's rate of population growth is a critical variable in any health workforce planning that seeks to meet minimum thresholds for health worker density. As an example, a country with a population of 10 million in 2020 requires 23,000 health workers to meet the threshold health worker density ratio. If the population grows at a rate of 2.4%, it will require an additional 53,360 health workers to meet the threshold 50 years later. This corresponds to more than a 200% increase over the number required (23,000) in the year 2020. Conversely, decreases in the annual rate of population growth can result in fewer additional health workers needed to reach the threshold health worker density ratio. A decrease can occur due to several factors including changes in fertility rates and use of contraception, increased mortality, etc. Because these rates don't change in a steady or predictable fashion, including these variables in models of workforce planning is difficult.

> *In 2019, the Association of American Medical Colleges (AAMC) projected a shortage of up to 121,900 physicians by 2032 including a shortage of up to 55,200 primary care physicians and approximately 67,000 specialists. (113)*

Catastrophic events such as the COVID-19 pandemic, although rare, highlight the unpredictability of the calculations of health care workforce sufficiency. Events of similar nature, albeit smaller magnitude, occur sometimes at the local level where outbreaks of infectious diseases for example can occur within a school district or a county leading to an increase in demand that could be temporary.

Geographical factors are not usually taken into account either. Due to the variable distribution of Hispanics in different regions, this type of planning "dilutes" the unmet need which is much higher in areas with high concentration of Hispanics (see section on maldistribution). Thus, a proper assessment of supply and demand must be conducted not only at the national level, but also regionally and locally. The temporal evolution of these regional differences must be taken into account as well.

During the signing of the Millennium Development goals (MDGs) in 2000, the WHO estimated that countries with less than 23 healthcare professionals (physicians, nurses and midwives) per 10,000 population would be unlikely to achieve adequate coverage rates for the key primary healthcare interventions prioritized by that initiative including: to eradicate extreme poverty and hunger, improve maternal health, to combat HIV/AIDS, malaria, and other diseases; among others.

By this measure, one could argue, as many others have, that there is a severe shortage of Hispanic physicians to cover for primary care interventions among the Hispanic population.

Is healthcare worker density sufficient to determine shortage and surplus of healthcare providers by race and ethnicity?

While overall physician shortage is strongly influenced by demographics (e.g. the fact that life expectancy has increased and baby boomers are aging and entering Medicare programs in record numbers [114]), when it comes to estimation of demand by race, **to say that more Hispanic physicians are needed simply because the worker density is low or because the number of Hispanics in the U.S. is growing is very simplistic. Even though this is a major driver of increased demand, it is**

evidently not reasonable to assume that only Hispanic physicians can care for Hispanic patients.

When people say that more physicians of a specific race/ethnicity are needed, that does not mean that minority professionals should only care for minority populations. **The importance of this statement is instead around improving the quality of care of minority patients by offering health care in their own language and by taking their cultural aspects into consideration.**

The primary objective of health workforce planning exercises is to balance supply and demand of healthcare providers in the short and long term. The amount of money allocated to workforce planning and the methodologies used vary in different geographies, but the interest in the process has increased over time due to changes in the population demographics. For example, longer life expectancies and increased health care use by the elderly and by low-income families through social security. Workforce planning informs and supports policy decisions and ensures adequate access to health care for the population.

Workforce planning models that help estimate the future demand do not typically take racial imbalances into account. Instead, the focus is on "replacement needs" based on the number of physicians graduating and retiring at a specific age. This assumes that the system is in balance as long as a sufficient number of new graduates is available to replace physicians leaving the workforce.

SUPPLY

- Number of Medical School graduates*: admission and drop-out rates, post-graduate training
- Number of immigrating professionals
- Workers coming back after leave of absence

- Retirement and pre-retirement attrition including emigration, change of career, etc.
- Remuneration: willingness of trained staff to accept pay and conditions
- Mortality
- Emigration

DEMAND

- Changes over time in the size of the population by age and sex, fertility rates, birth and death rates, immigration
- Current and possible future use of healthcare services by segments of the population (age, sex, race/ethnicity)

- Morbidity patterns and burden of different disaesses and risk factors
- "Plasticity" of services: adjustment of services according to local practices and multidisciplinary patient management

- Changes in Expenditure: amount of resources available to pay for health care, salaries, benefits, willingness, to pay for healthcare, etc

FIGURE 32. HEALTHCARE WORKER DRIVERS FOR SUPPLY AND DEMAND. MODIFIED FROM [124] [125] [126]. ONE OF THE MOST IMPORTANT DRIVERS OF HEALTH WORKFORCE SUPPLY IS THE NUMBER OF MEDICAL SCHOOL GRADUATES.

Knowing that the number of medical school graduates is one of the key drivers of health workforce inflows, the inequality in the number of Hispanic graduates in comparison with graduates from other races and ethnicities is a major issue. Another issue is that the definition of shortage is unclear. Shortages have been estimated using the multiple different metrics listed in **Box 2**.

BOX 2. VARIABLES COMMONLY USED TO DEFINE PHYSICIAN SHORTAGES

Variables commonly used to define physician shortages

Vacancy rates from hospital surveys- Average length of time to fill posts or data on hospital vacancies

Comparison to a benchmark- Gap between current physician- to- population ratio and a benchmark or target.

Patient focused measures- Difficulties finding physicians or waiting time to get appointments

Size of the population with poor health- To estimate demand among those most in need

Furthermore, workforce planning typically assumes that there is no current shortage or surplus of physicians. However, as I explained when I described the White-Hispanic gap in standardized test scores, the starting point is already uneven. The starting numbers for healthcare providers correspond to census data without any of the variables listed above such as geography and racial imbalances taken into account.

Some people believe that a good way to address this issue is by comparing local shortages with a benchmark. However, the proper benchmark is unknown, and it does not apply to all populations, i.e. what is an appropriate benchmark for one race (e.g. White), may not apply to other races (e.g. Hispanics) precisely due to the starting inequalities. The main advantage of using a benchmark is to plan for a target in which all races have same access to care. However, as mentioned before, Hispanic physicians should not be restricted to treat Hispanic patients.

Underrepresentation or maldistribution

Geographic maldistribution of physicians is another major factor associated with insufficient access to health care. Instead of a shortage of healthcare providers, some analysts have shown that there is a strong concentration of certain medical specialties in discrete areas of the country. [115] In an analysis of non-federal primary care physicians under the age of 75, a physician surplus was only observed in discrete areas of the country. [116]

In a retrospective cohort study using 2012 data from the American Medical Association (AMA) Physician Masterfile, [117] researchers looked at the racial and ethnic composition as well as practice locations of a cohort of more than 140,000 primary care physicians who graduated from medical schools in or after 1980, when race and ethnicity started to be systematically collected. The study also analyzed the population access to primary health care.

In their cohort, 6.8% (or 10,064) physicians were Black, 5.9% (or 8,697) Hispanic, 72.5% (107,222) White, and 2.9% (or 4,314) other or unknown race/ethnicity. As expected, the diversity of this cohort of physicians did not reflect the diversity of the U.S. population at the time of the study. Accessibility to care was defined as the number of primary care physicians available per 10,000 population.

The study reports several important findings some of which the authors very effectively illustrate in a map [117] and that I will summarize here:

1. Hispanic physicians practice in greater numbers than White primary care physicians in Primary Care Health Professional Shortage Areas (HPSA), Medically Underserved Areas/Populations (MUA/P), and rural areas. This was true even after excluding international medical graduates who represent more than 20% of the primary care physician population, at least in some geographies.

2. There are significant differences in geographic distribution and diversity of primary care specialties.

3. Family medicine was the least diverse and internal medicine the most diverse specialty.

4. Florida, Southern Texas, New Mexico, central Colorado, Arizona, California, Washington, and Puerto Rico are the states most affected for primary care accessibility by the presence of Hispanic primary care physicians. [117]

Interestingly, when looking at other maps on physician distribution created by the AAMC using data from the AAMC's 2013 Minority Physician Database, which I encourage you to review, it is immediately obvious that **the number of Hispanic physicians is so low, that clear differences from state to state are difficult to discern, in comparison to those differences in distribution of the White or the Black healthcare workforce**. With the exception of Puerto Rico, New Mexico, Florida, Texas, California and Arizona, the percentage of physicians of Hispanic origin is less than 5% in all other states in the U.S. In fact, it is lower than 4% in most states.

Percentage of physicians practicing in underserved areas, selected states

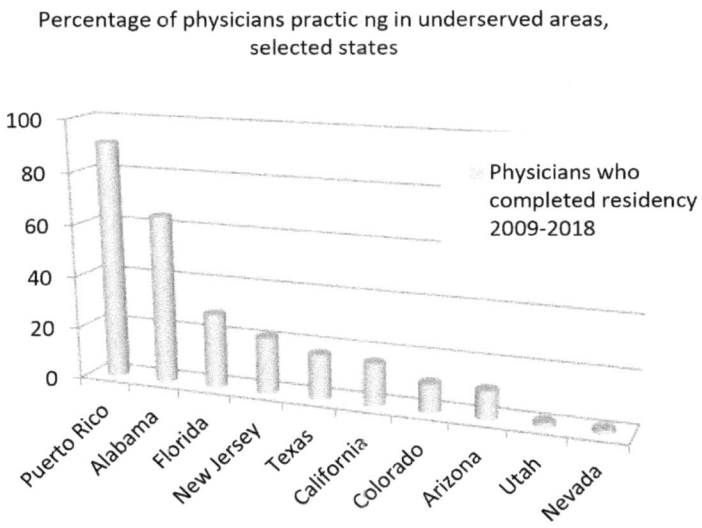

FIGURE 33. PHYSICIANS PRACTICING IN UNDERSERVED AREAS, BY STATE. (MORE THAN HALF (54.6%) OF THE INDIVIDUALS WHO COMPLETED THEIR RESIDENCY TRAINING FROM 2009 THROUGH 2018 ARE PRACTICING IN THE STATE WHERE THEY DID THEIR RESIDENCY TRAINING.)

In a survey of physicians in California, it was found that the supply of physicians was inversely associated with the proportion of Black and Hispanic residents, and that Hispanic physicians were two times more likely than White physicians to practice in communities with high proportions of Hispanic residents and in areas with fewer primary care physicians per capita. [118]

Another study reported a ratio of Latino resident physicians to the Latino population in the four states with the largest Latino populations: California, Texas, Florida, and New York between 2001 and 2017. By 2011, the national average was 36.6 residents and fellows per 100,000. California and New York had the lowest and highest rates respectively at 5.4 and 28.4 residents and fellows per 100,000 Latino population. Texas and Florida fell somewhere in between. [119] As these studies show, minority areas tend to face shortages of physicians, yet non-White physicians are disproportionately more likely to serve in these communities.

Finally, an average of 23.3% of physicians who completed their residency training between 2009 and 2018, practice in Medically Underserved Areas across all 50 states, regardless of where they completed residency training.

Percent of need met health professional shortage areas, 2019

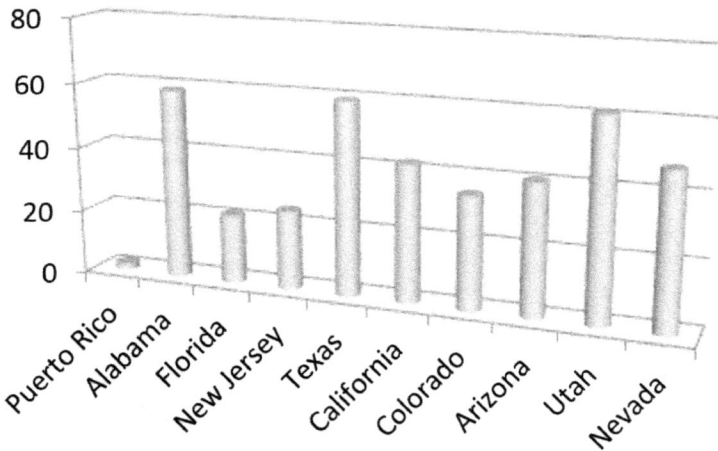

FIGURE 34. PERCENT OF NEED MET HEALTH PROFESSIONAL SHORTAGE AREAS, 2019

However, as shown in Figure 33, variability is high across states. One consideration is that states have different numbers of areas designated as Medically Underserved Areas and thus these numbers are relative. The HRSA quantifies the "percent of need met" by dividing the number of primary care physicians available to serve the population of an area, by the number of physicians that would be necessary to eliminate the designation of health professional shortage areas. According to that measure, only 1.92% of the need was met in Puerto Rico and close to 60% of the need met in Utah in 2019, as shown in Figure 34.

More Hispanic physicians obtain financial a d that comes with obligations to work in underserved areas. This may confound conclusions that URM practice more in underserved areas.

Interventions

Some of the information presented in this book is incontrovertible. The data on the size of the Hispanic population and the prevalence of Spanish as the most commonly spoken language in the U.S. other than English are based on sound data. However, other topics related

to policy or those recently debated, such as whether attempts to increase diversity in healthcare education result in unfair selection of under qualified candidates, are complex and controversial issues that I will not pretend to be able to appropriately address. As in all chapters, I provide a short summary in the section below, accompanied with extensive references for those interested in reading more about these topics.

Modifying trends in educational attainment can only take place over long periods of time and requires both recognition of the importance of education and the involvement of multiple areas of society beyond just the education community.

Meaningful change requires at least two elements (1) Collaboration between organizations and institutions committed to racial and ethnic diversity in the health professions, and (2) Funding to execute corrective measures, to support research on the barriers to improving diversity and inclusion, and to evaluate outcomes of strategies that address risk factors for low educational attainment at all points along the educational continuum—especially in early stages where the disparities begin. Change also requires commitment by leadership, changes in institutional policies and mission statements, as well as grassroots activism among students. [120-122]

In their policy series, the Latino Policy and Politics Initiative from UCLA proposes a six-item strategy to help address the shortfall in Latino resident physicians [119] that includes:

1. increasing medical school admissions for Latinos,
2. retaining MD graduates who attend out-of-state medical schools,
3. implementing K-12 programs to encourage students to pursue careers in medicine,
4. expanding MD programs,
5. emphasizing the need for care in underserved communities,
6. increasing the number of international medical graduates, and increasing the number of residency slots in order to expand training in settings serving medically and linguistically underserved communities.

Established in 2003, the Sullivan Commission on Diversity in the Healthcare Workforce has the goal of making policy recommendations designed to bring about systemic changes that would address the scarcity of minorities in the health professions. The Commission seeks to address the under-enrollment of minorities in health professions education, in line with the recommendation by the Institute of Medicine to increase the number of minority health professionals as a key strategy to eliminate health disparities. [123] After a series of six field hearings across the country with 140 participants from the health, education, religion and business communities, the Sullivan Commission published the report entitled: "Missing Persons: Minorities in the Health Professions" [124], which emphasizes the importance of diversity in the health professions and the urgency for action aimed at correcting the current disparities in medical education. The report highlights three core principles considered essential to achieving their mission:

1. **To increase diversity in the health professions, the culture of health professions schools must change**. Cultural changes occurring in our society as a consequence of the changes in demographics must be reflected in the culture of medical schools around the country.

2. **New and nontraditional paths to the health professions should be explored**. The K-12 educational system must improve. The current path for most health professions requires 10-12 years of education.

3. **Commitments must be at the highest levels**. Institutional leaders must be supportive of the changes. Without leadership support, there can be no meaningful and long-lasting change. [124]

Interventions at the college level seem to be effective at increasing the entrance to medical school. Programs like the Minority Medical Education program have demonstrated that a 6-week program significantly increased the probability of acceptance to medical school. Interventions to support minority student performance in college gateway courses is also beneficial. [92]

Finally, the demographic composition of each school and institution should not only determined by the willingness of the school leadership to address diversity issues, but also by the demographic composition of the local community, the demographics of the faculty, the cost and affiliations of the school, among other factors. [125]

A few examples of schools and institutions that have programs in place aimed at closing the gap among ethnic and racial groups, or that have already made strides toward more diverse membership and whose learnings could be shared are:

1. The University of California which reported enrollment of 32.6% Latinos in 2016. This number went up to 34% by 2018, which was considered the most diverse freshman class ever for UC. [126] Their post baccalaureate premedical programs seem to result in an increase in the number of medical school matriculants from disadvantaged and underrepresented groups. [127]

2. Harvard University Class of 2020, which is the school's most diverse class yet with 12% Latinos enrolled. [128]

3. Premedical Honors programs such as the Baylor/Rice program, which according to their website provides promising students underrepresented in medicine with educational and practical experiences to enhance their competitiveness in the medical school admissions process. Students receive conditional acceptance. Tuition and other costs are paid for by the program.

4. The minority recruitment and retention program at Duke University and the Multicultural Resource Center at UCSF.

5. The Stanford Medical Youth Science Program (SMYP), which was a 5-week summer program for low-income students from 20 California counties, as well as other summer educational programs for minority students led by individual US medical schools or consortia of medical schools. [129, 130]

6. Recommendations for improving pipeline programs have been published using examples from the University of Nebraska Medical Center. [131, 132]

7. The Diverse Surgeons Initiative (DSI) which trains URM residents on surgical skills and clinical knowledge, but also provides mentorship and assists residents in attaining fellowships. [133]

It has been proposed that increasing medical school enrollment would address the physician shortage. However, as I've shown here, medical school enrollment has continued to grow not only for Hispanics but for all races/ethnicities (up 30% since 2002).

It has also been proposed that the Medicare cap has prevented many of those medical school graduates from finding places to continue their training, which leads to the conclusion that physician shortages could not be addressed by simply increasing access to medical schools, unless a sufficient number of training programs are available after graduation. [134] However, according to a study using 20 years of residency data, in spite of the implementation of Medicare caps in 1997, the number of first-year residency positions has increased at the same rate since 2003 as it did before the introduction of the caps. [135] This suggests that increasing the number of physicians does not depend on additional federal funding. In fact, some reports suggest that a sufficient number of first-year ACGME-accredited training positions have been created to accommodate the increased number of medical school graduates. [136] In their 2018 press release, the National Resident Matching Program stated that the Main Residency Match had been the largest in NRMP history with a record-high 37,103 applicants submitting program choices for 33,167 positions, the most ever offered. The number of first-year (PGY-1) positions available increased by 1,383 from 30,232 the previous year of 2017.

Clearly this issue is more complex than just the number of graduates or the number of residency slots. As I have shown throughout this chapter, racial and ethnic underrepresentation begins early and continues all throughout the educational journey.

Apart from addressing issues such as maldistribution, the most important nationwide initiative is the affirmative action act, which I will briefly discuss next.

Affirmative action

Out of all policies mentioned above, affirmative action deserves separate consideration because despite being continuously controversial, it is frequently cited as the main means to increase diversity in higher education. In summary, affirmative action can be defined as a proactive effort to ensure that people are not discriminated against on the basis of their gender or their ethnic group. It goes beyond equal opportunity to allocating resources to identify, prevent and correct discrimination.

> *"I am a product of affirmative action. I am the perfect affirmative action baby. I am Puerto Rican, born and raised in the south Bronx. My test scores were not comparable to my colleagues at Princeton and Yale. Not so far off so that I wasn't able to succeed at those institutions."*
> *− Sonia Sotomayor*

Affirmative action can be understood in multiple ways and a detailed discussion on the topic is beyond the scope of this book. I encourage those interested in the topic to read the following article by Crosby et al. [137]

Affirmative action seeks to improve opportunities for underrepresented or disadvantaged groups, especially in relation to employment and education. The mechanisms utilized for this purpose include a) financial support to help minorities gain access to higher education, b) hiring practices that require the inclusion of diverse candidates for job openings, c) requirements that a minimum percentage of qualified professionals from varying ethnicities and genders are employed in order for those institutions to be eligible for funding.

One of the aspects of affirmative action that is relevant to this book is its influence on higher education, which has been the cause of significant controversy. The main goal of affirmative action plans in higher education is to increase diversity. Critics of affirmative action argue (1) that the program could lead to the admission of less qualified candidates (reverse discrimination), (2) that the Constitution protects citizens of all races equally, and (3) that the program has had minimal impact and, therefore, the cost does not justify the outcome.

Quantitative data on the impact of affirmative action plans on diversity in higher education has only recently been generated. Publications such as the acclaimed book by the presidents of Harvard and Princeton universities in the late 1990s, [138] not only showed a significant increase in diversity in admissions as a consequence of affirmative action plans, but also that minority students being admitted were graduating at the same rate as White students.

However, one aspect highlighted by Crosby et al, is a finding reported by Sander in a 2004 paper in which it was concluded that race-sensitive admission policies have resulted in fewer African American students graduating from law school in top-tier schools and passing the bar exam, possibly because it's better for them to be at the top of the class in a low-tier school than it is to be at the bottom of the class in a high-tier school.

This is an interesting point that has been raised by Malcolm Gladwell in his book David and Goliath. I am only bringing this up here because it appears to have received quite a lot of publicity, to the extent that one of the medical school students that I recently interviewed appeared to be convinced that if he was able to enter a high-tier medical school in the North-East, his chances of doing well were much lower than his white counterparts'.

Using several famous examples such as the story of David and Goliath, and that of painters such as Van Gogh and his contemporary impressionists, Gladwell tries to make the point that "there are times and places when it's better to be a little fish in a big pond than a big fish in a little pond because the apparent disadvantage of being an outsider in a marginal world turns out not to be a disadvantage at all." [139] Even if the examples provided in his book are merely illustrative and his conclusions are derived from interpretation, they are in line with the findings of some studies on the impact of the environment and self-judgment on academic achievement.

Once admitted to medical school, minority students admitted through affirmative action programs have the same probability to graduate as non-minority students regardless of their test scores and GPA at the time of enrollment.

As Crosby and colleagues state in their review article, there are numerous reasons why this assumption that disadvantaged students don't have an equal chance to succeed in top-ranked schools cannot be supported by data and can certainly not be generalized. However, there is something to be said about the overall psychological impact of the culture of certain schools that can be a difficult adjustment for students coming from different environments.

This topic has been addressed in another interesting book by Anthony Abraham Jack, who highlights the fact that admission does not equal inclusion. In his book, he qualifies students as double-disadvantaged when they come from local neighborhood schools that are likely segregated and overcrowded with limited resources and often high rates of violence. These students are unfamiliar with elite prep schools. In contrast, "privileged poor" students who gain access to elite schools thanks to affirmative action programs have opportunities to study abroad, learn other languages or, at the very least, to become accustomed to navigating elite academic arenas, which increases their chances of success. [140]

As with many policies of this nature, affirmative action creates both positive and negative reactions. [141-144] In their paper, Crosby et al even review some of the known reasons behind differing attitudes towards it.

According to The Center for Equal Opportunity headed by Linda Chavez, [145] a conservative Hispanic who is well-known for her opposition to the affirmative action, a study sampling six medical schools revealed a dramatic difference in the odds of admission between African American applicants and, to a lesser degree Hispanic applicants, in comparison with White and Asian applicants, even when they had higher undergraduate grades and MCAT scores.

Recent changes in affirmative action policy in some states, such as those related to elimination of schools' ability to consider race and ethnicity as factors in admissions resulting from law suits, judicial decisions, and pressure from the current administration has resulted in decreases in enrollment of underrepresented minorities into medical schools and affected the successful completion of several affirmative action programs. [121, 146]

While some critics object to using federal funds to place students in elite schools instead of using those funds to improve public education, others focus on the idea that affirmative action plans give an unfair advantage to minorities. I won't confirm or deny this grave hypothesis because that debate appears to be impossible to settle. However, I do question why, if all these affirmative action plans have provided such a dramatic advantage to minorities, there is still such clear and widespread disparity? It is clear to me that the perceived advantage of affirmative action is not sufficient to compensate for the disparities. If the advantage granted through affirmative action was sufficient there would be no inequality between Hispanics and Whites in the healthcare workforce or in any other area.

A key message of this book is that affirmative action plans are still needed simply because racial discrimination still exists, and in an environment of increased pressure from the current administration to eliminate the consideration of race as a criterion for admissions, action must be taken to ensure equal opportunity for students of all races and ethnicities.

Key takeaways from chapter 3

1

Hispanic representation levels are below those for other minorities at all education levels. However, the number of Hispanic children enrolled in elementary education has increased over time, the number of Hispanics obtaining high school diplomas and going to college is at an all-time high, the dropout rate has decreased and the number of Hispanics obtaining a bachelor's degree has doubled in the last decade.

2

Disparities begin as early as kindergarten and it's been stated that the biggest impediment to a diverse healthcare workforce in the U.S. is the inability of primary education to meet the needs of minority and low income students.

3

Educational achievement, as measured by reading and science scores is lower among Hispanic students in the 4th, 8th and 12th grades and the White-Hispanic gap has generally not narrowed since the 1990s. It has been said that achievement scores have an inherent racial bias, but many other factors such as English proficiency are important. Because of the higher poverty levels among Hispanics and the higher rates of students with non-educated parents, Hispanics are less prepared for these tests, but this can be addressed by accessing free test preparation services.

4

While Asian Americans represent only slightly over 5% of the U.S. young adult population, they represent more than 20% of medical school applicants. In contrast, Hispanics represent more than 20% of the young adult population of the country, and only 6.5% of the medical school applicants. The number of White applicants mirrors their representation in the general population.

5

In spite of the challenges associated with the determination of the sufficiency of the workforce, by all existing measures there is a shortage of Hispanic physicians in the U.S.

6

Minority areas tend to face shortages of physicians, yet non-White physicians are disproportionately more likely to serve in these communities.

7

Meaningful change requires commitment by the leadership and changes in institutional policies and mission statements, grassroots activism among students and funding to execute corrective measures, support research on the barriers to improving diversity and inclusion, and to evaluate outcomes. K-12 education must improve.

Online resources for chapter 3

IF YOU ARE INTERESTED IN:

Information on the journey from Pre-Med Through Residency	https://students-residents.aamc.org/
Cost of Medical School and financial aid	https://store.aamc.org/medical-student-education-debt-costs-and-loan-repayment-fact-card-2019-pdf.html https://aamcfinancialwellness.com/index.cfm and visit the AAMC YouTube channel
How to pay for Medical School	https://students-residents.aamc.org/financial-aid/article/5-things-pay-for-med-school/
Scholarships, Health Careers Opportunities and Primary care residency training in: Family Medicine Internal Medicine Pediatrics Internal Medicine-Pediatrics Obstetrics and Gynecology	Health Careers Opportunities Program and the Center of Excellence Program BHW Funding Opportunities Health Careers Opportunity Program: The National HCOP Academies Teaching Health Center Graduate Medical Education (THCGME) Program

https://bhw.hrsa.gov/grants/
medicine/thcgme
https://www.hrsa.gov/grants/find-
funding/HRSA-20-011

Scholarships https://bhw.hrsa.gov/
loans-scholarships/nhsc
The National Health Service Corps
(NHSC) awards scholarships and loan
repayment to primary care providers
in eligible disciplines https://nhsc.
hrsa.gov/scholarships/index.html

For Hispanics:
https://www.colgatepalmolive.com/
en-us/core-values/community-
responsibility/make-the-u

Diverse Medical Scholars Program
includes renewal scholarships
for Med School students:
https://nmfonline.org/about-
our-scholarships-and-awards/
service-learning-programs/united-
health-foundationnmf-diverse-
medical-scholars-program/

https://nmf.fluidreview.com/

Thurgood Marshall College Fund:
https://tmcf.org/students-alumni/
scholarships/open-scholarships/

The Jackie Robinson foundation:
https://www.jackierobinson.org/
apply/applicants/

	TYLENOL® Future Care Scholarship https://www.tylenol.com/news/scholarship
	Herbert W. Nickens Medical Student Scholarships https://www.aamc.org/what-we-do/aamc-awards/nickens-medical-student-scholarships
Resources for aspiring and current Medical School students	American Academy of Family Physicians https://www.aafp.org/home.html https://www.aafp.org/medical-school-residency.html
	Physicians of tomorrow awards: $10,000 scholarship for Med School students: https://www.ama-assn.org/about/awards/physicians-tomorrow-awards
Free help to prepare for MCAT	https://www.khanacademy.org/test-prep/mcat
Free help to prepare for SAT	https://www.khanacademy.org/test-prep/sat
The Casper® test	https://takecasper.com/test-prep/

Getting more resources because you believe that your community is experiencing a shortage of healthcare professionals and want to apply for shortage designation	https://bhw.hrsa.gov/shortage-designation/what-is-shortage-designation
Internship opportunities for URM students and programs to address the serious shortage of Latino physicians and other healthcare professionals in the area	http://www.fresno.ucsf.edu/latino-center-for-medical-education-and-research/admissions-hcop/ Latino Center for Medical Education and Research. Fresno https://www.fresno.ucsf.edu/latino-center-for-medical-education-and-research/ Gateway to higher Education programs NYC and Mount Sinai http://www.gateway.cuny.edu/about-gateway/timeline-boxes/index.html Gateway to Higher Education (program) The Stanford Medical Youth Science Program (SMYP) https://smysp.spcs.stanford.edu/about
Webinars on tools for measuring equality, improving care for diverse populations	The Disparities Solutions Center https://mghdisparitiessolutions.org/ podcast that can be accessed directly here: https://anchor.fm/disparitiessolutions

Electronic Residency Application Service (ERAS) Data	https://www.aamc.org/data/facts/eras/
Data on demographics of Medical School applicants, residents and medical school faculty. Current data on diversity in Medicine, among others	Association of American Medical Colleges https://www.aamc.org/data
Publications related to the underrepresentation of minorities in specific medical specialties	[147-152]
Data from early childhood through postsecondary education.	U.S. Department of Education. National Center for Education Statistics (NCES) NCES obtains consistent information from specified nationally representative groups of individuals and institutions. Resources available, include the data lab which can be used to generate tables and figures
Early Care and Education	The Hispanic Research Center. Interactive data tool https://www.hispanicresearchcenter.org/

	https://www.hispanicresearchcenter.org/research-resources/data-tool-early-care-and-education-search-and-decision-making/ https://www.hispanicresearchcenter.org/research-resources/data-tool-families-utilization-of-early-care-and-education/
Data on standardized test results	The NAEP National Assessment of educational progress provides per year State comparisons regarding test scores
Laws related to standardized testing including the No Child Left Behind and the newer Every Student Succeeds Act	U.S. Department of Education https://www.ed.gov/essa
Colleges with the highest number of Hispanic students	10 Colleges With the Most Hispanic Students
Hub of research to improve the lives of Hispanics across three areas economics, family structure, and early childcare and education.	The National Research Center on Hispanic Children & Families (Center) http://www.hispanicresearchcenter.org/focus-areas/#early-care-and-education
Data on children and families child well-being in the United States	Kids Count KIDS COUNT Data Book https://datacenter.kidscount.org/

Data on leading civil rights indicators related to access and barriers to educational opportunity at the early childhood through grade 12 levels.	Department of Education, Office for Civil Rights Office for Civil Rights The CRDC collects Annual report: https://www2.ed.gov/about/offices/list/ocr/congress.html To file a complaint with the office for Civil Rights: https://www2.ed.gov/about/offices/list/ocr/docs/howto.html?src=rt
Data on STEM students	National Center for Science and Engineering Statistics https://ncses.nsf.gov/pubs/nsf19304/digest/field-of-degree-minorities#hispanic-or-latino-graduates https://ncses.nsf.gov/pubs/nsf19304/
Health Workforce Analysis-HRSA	The National Center for Health Workforce Analysis (NCHWA) is the national resource for health workforce research, information, and data. The NCHWA conducts workforce analysis in various healthcare occupations and performance metrics and evaluations of health workforce training and education programs.

Health Workforce Analysis-North Carolina University Shep Center's forecasting tool.

This model forecasts utilization instead of need or demand, and it takes into account a number of variables including future number of physician visits for a population in a specific geographic area by health condition and in different medical settings (e.g. doctors' offices and hospital and emergency settings). [153] To my knowledge, the variable of race/ethnicity in the supply model is not taken into account which prevents the use of this very dynamic model to estimate shortage or surplus of Hispanic doctors specifically.

CHAPTER FOUR

EDUCATIONAL ATTAINMENT BEYOND THE NUMBERS

Why is there a shortage of Hispanic physicians in the U.S.?

"Health equity targets for underserved population groups will remain elusive if they do not consider how health workers can be effectively recruited and retained to work among them."
– World Health Report 2008

"Until we get equality in education, we will not have an equal society"
– Sonia Sotomayor, U.S. Supreme Court Justice

ANA MARIA FACES MULTIPLE RISKS FOR EDUCATIONAL ATTAINMENT

Ana Maria says, "I keep hearing, 'Your parents are already struggling to pay for your sister's treatments. How could they help you with college? How can you devote enough time to school when you have to care for your younger siblings? Who would take care of them if you left?' When I ask for help, these are the questions people keep asking me!"

Ana Maria felt marginalized from the early days of school. Despite her efforts to impress her teachers, she was constantly discouraged by everyone around her. She kept dreaming about going to medical school and she constantly sought mentorship and support, but this often seemed to be lacking.

This part of Ana Maria's story illustrates a common theme among Hispanics in the U.S. In addition to the high cost of medical school that her parents could not possibly help with, she has all the risk factors associated with low educational attainment. Poverty, parents with low level of education, a household where Spanish is spoken, and she attends a segregated school with high dropout rates and lack of mentorship and teacher support. [82, 154]

The educational journey

Depicted in the figure below is the journey of a student throughout the pipeline, highlighting some of the barriers for success that will be discussed in this chapter.

When compared with White students, racial and ethnic minority students receive a K-12 education of measurably lower quality, score lower on standardized tests, and are less likely to complete high school.

In elementary and secondary school, one key issue is the quality of the educational programs, which is very heterogeneous nationwide and of lesser quality for schools with high numbers of Hispanic students and English language learners.

In high school, key factors include high dropout rates and disparities associated with standardized tests. Poverty and other circumstances described in the next chapter prevent many students from applying to college in the first place. Among those that do apply, many are rejected are unable to attend due to financial constraints, or are not adequately prepared and may drop out. At the residency level, some of the most important issues are lack of funding, maldistribution and discrimination.

Risk factors for low educational attainment among Hispanics

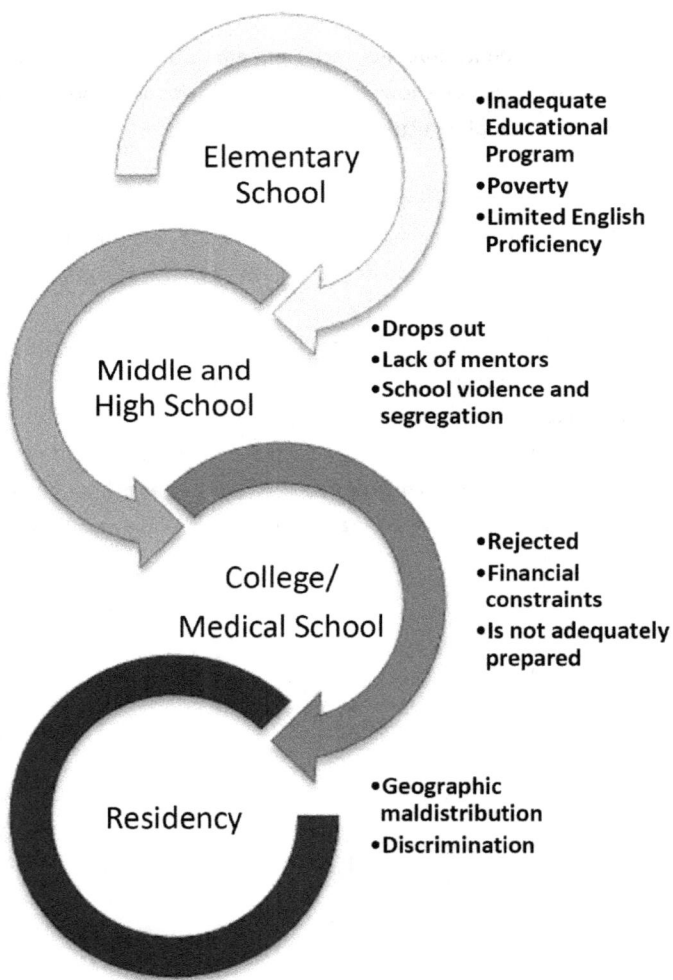

- Inadequate Educational Program
- Poverty
- Limited English Proficiency

Elementary School

- Drops out
- Lack of mentors
- School violence and segregation

Middle and High School

- Rejected
- Financial constraints
- Is not adequately prepared

College/ Medical School

- Geographic maldistribution
- Discrimination

Residency

FIGURE 35. THE EDUCATIONAL JOURNEY, FROM ELEMENTARY SCHOOL TO RESIDENCY

A study conducted by Salud America estimated that as many as 78% of Hispanic children suffer from an adverse event in childhood, including poverty, abuse, neglect, divorce, among others. Exposure to more than one of these risk factors has a cumulative effect on long-term outcomes, and this is, of course, true not only for Hispanic children. The Fragile Families and Child Wellbeing Study was a national birth cohort including approximately 25% Hispanic children. It showed that exposure to 3 or more adverse childhood experiences results in below-average math, language and literacy skills, as well as attention problems and aggression in kindergarten.

Figure 36 depicts some of the most important risk factors for low educational attainment.

Many scholars have proposed that the differences in formal education enrollment are primarily due to differences in family income. Hispanic children often live in two-parent households with parents who are employed, but the income of Hispanic families is approximately 60% that of White families. [155-157] These differences would continue to apply to the same children over time and into adolescence and adulthood. However, separating poverty from any other individual risk factor for low educational attainment is nearly impossible. [158] For example, one risk factor for poor academic achievement is being born to undereducated parents, but undereducated parents are more likely to also be low income earners.

The research around the critical importance of Pre-K education in long-term outcomes is so clear that numerous programs have been put in place to support Pre-K education nationwide. [159] However, few studies have evaluated the impact of Early Childhood Education (ECE) or specific early childhood home environments on educational outcomes in adulthood. [160, 161] Some have found a correlation between early life environment and long-term outcomes by dropout rates and academic achievement, [161-163] but rigorous longitudinal research looking at different races and ethnicities is lacking. [160] This makes it difficult to conclude that differences in ECE between Hispanic and non-Hispanic children living in the U.S. are directly or indirectly responsible for their low educational attainment later in life.

Because of the variability in the design and objectives of different ECE programs, it is difficult to precisely determine their long-term impact. Thus, studies that examine long-term outcomes need to adjust for such factors as program objectives, duration, intensity, program and teacher quality, and many other factors. Most systematic studies of the impact of ECE programs have concluded that enrollment in "any" program does not equal better outcomes. High quality, intensive programs, characterized by low group sizes, adequate child-staff ratios, and high teacher qualifications, are needed. [164]

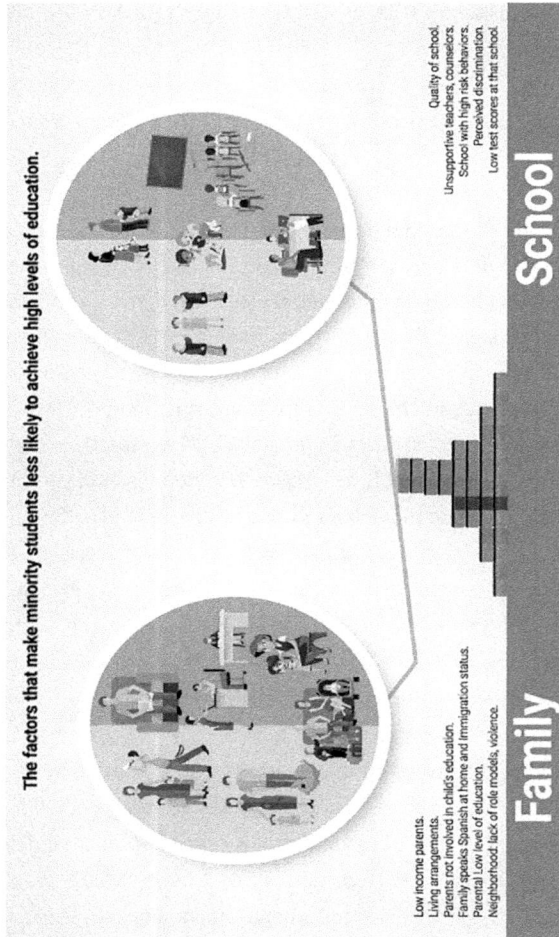

FIGURE 36. RISK FACTORS FOR LOW EDUCATIONAL ATTAINMENT

The objective of this chapter is therefore not to draw any direct conclusions regarding the association between ECE and long-term outcomes such as medical school enrollment rates, but to describe the similarities and differences between Hispanics and other racial and ethnic groups, particularly Blacks and Whites throughout the educational journey from ECE through college and beyond. I will also try not to focus only on deficits, but also on strengths around Hispanic upbringing in relationship to educational attainment. The "Status and Trends in the Education of Racial and Ethnic Groups" latest report published in February of 2019 is a great resource for detailed information on student challenges by racial and ethnic background in the U.S. [165]

Poverty and parental level of education

In the Early Childhood Longitudinal Study (ECLS), poverty status was based on household income below poverty thresholds defined by the U.S. census bureau. **Hispanics have an official poverty rate of 17.6% in 2018 (representing 10.5 million people),** significantly higher than the overall U.S. poverty rate of 11.8% and the White poverty rate of 10.8% (15.7 million people).

Eight key findings from the available demographic data:

1. Children's social class is one of the most significant predictors of their educational success. In 2010, over half of children in the lowest socioeconomic status quartile (50.4%) were Hispanic (compared to 39.8% in 1998).
2. Coming from a low-income family is a significant risk for scoring low in reading, mathematics and science as early as kindergarten. Hispanic men earn 66 cents for every dollar earned by White men in 2016. Hispanic women earn 69 cents on the dollar.

3. Students who live in poverty and who don't have a parent who completed high school, tend to score lower in science, math and reading during the first four years of school, compared to students who don't have these risk factors. Importantly, this starts early in life. The percentage of first-time kindergartners who have both risk factors is higher for Hispanic students (15%) than for other races, e.g. Blacks 8%, Whites 1%.

4. Children who grow up in poverty have limited access to healthy food, high-quality educational programs and recreation spaces[166] that are all associated with better long-term outcomes. [167] Limited access to healthful food can lead to either malnutrition, which is associated with poor school outcomes, or possibly also to obesity. [168] Hispanic children are more likely to become overweight before starting elementary school than children of other ethnic groups [169] and to be less physically active, which is also associated with poor outcomes. [170]

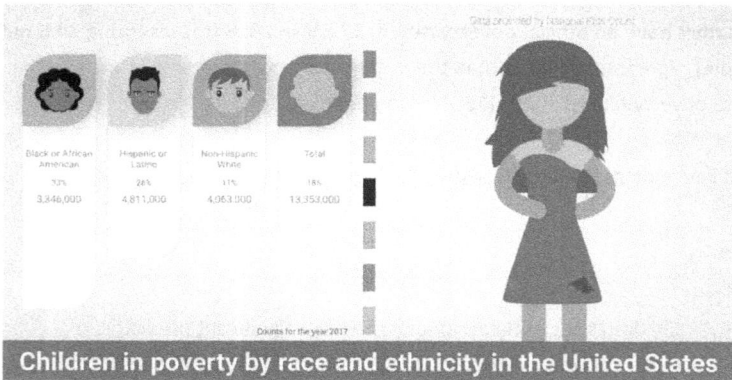

Children in poverty by race and ethnicity in the United States

FIGURE 37. THE PERCENTAGE OF CHILDREN UNDER AGE 18 LIVING IN POVERTY, BY PARENTS' HIGHEST LEVEL OF EDUCATIONAL ATTAINMENT, CHILD'S RACE/ETHNICITY, 2017

5. The percentage of Hispanic children in poverty was 26% and 11% for Whites, in 2018. [1,2]

6. Neighborhood economic hardship has been reported to be a significant predictor of children's lower academic outcomes. [171]

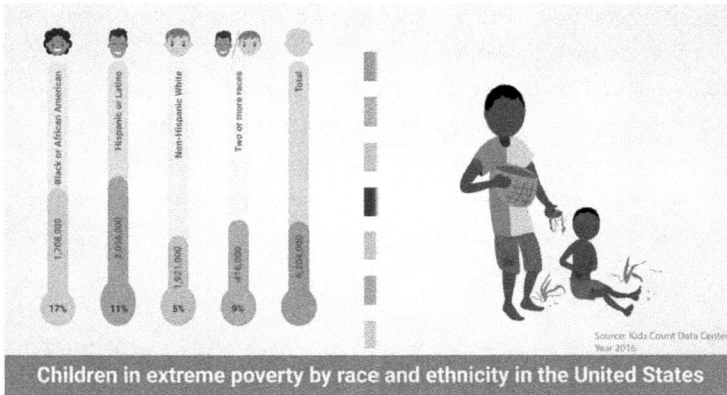

Children in extreme poverty by race and ethnicity in the United States

FIGURE 38. CHILDREN IN EXTREME POVERTY BY RACE AND ETHNICITY

7. In 2016, the percentage of children under age 18 who lived in households without a parent who had completed high school was higher for Hispanic children (26%) than for White (4%). 6% of Hispanic versus only 1% of White kindergartners did not have a parent who completed high school.

8. In an AAMC report from 2018, the authors conclude that three-quarters of medical school matriculants come from the top two household-income quintiles. The top quintiles correspond to incomes of $74,870- $121,018 and ≥$121,019- ≥$225,251. In fact, more than one third of all U.S. medical school first-year students in this analysis

1. Children in poverty = children under age 18 who live in families with incomes below the federal poverty level
2. This percentage varied significantly among Hispanic subgroups and geographic locations.

came from families in highest-income quintile that comprises the top 5% of U.S. households (≥$225,251). This distribution hasn't changed in three decades. [172]

9. How students pay for higher education varies considerably by race and ethnicity, especially in terms of who borrows and who leaves college with high levels of student loan debt. Asian and Hispanic students are the least likely to borrow.

10. Admission requirements are in place to ensure that only the most qualified candidates are accepted. However, meeting those requirements means going through a process that is too costly financially and emotionally for low income students without a strong support network.

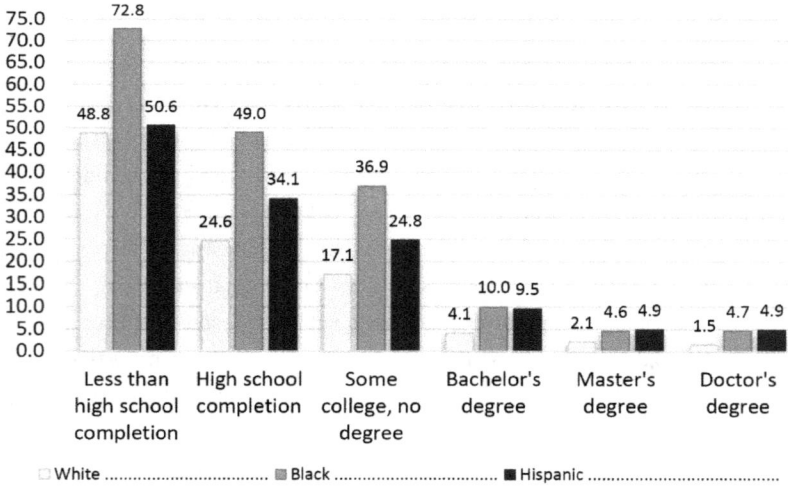

The percentage of children under age 18 living in poverty is higher if the parents have low educational attainment

FIGURE 39. CHILDREN IN EXTREME POVERTY BY PARENTAL LEVEL OF EDUCATION

Most available data supports the intuitive assumption that children who grow up in stable, low-conflict, two-parent families have a higher probability of faring better than children growing up in other family types. Parental conflict is associated with children's poorer academic achievement, increased substance use, and higher risk of dropping out of high school. [173]

However, the relationships are complex because the definitions are not clear cut. For example, the definition of a "low-conflict" and "high-conflict" marriage and the study of their relationship to children's outcomes are difficult. Aspects such as how often disagreements become violent, how often parents reach resolutions and how to measure psychological impact of even minimal conflict are not usually taken into account in most studies.

The data on living arrangements and parental conflict by race and ethnicity is somewhat controversial. It has been stated that numbers are inflated due to inaccurate self-reporting rates associated issues such as tax advantages for single mothers. Yet, one could argue that a family in which the mother miss-reports living arrangements due to poverty or relationship dysfunction is likely to be a high-risk family in terms of the children's outcomes.

On the other hand, some studies have found that Hispanic children may have an advantage in several aspects of early life environments. [160, 174] For example, Hispanic children often live in relatively stable two-parent households with parents who are steadily employed, which can be perceived as an advantage at least when comparing with children of other races and ethnicities, particularly Black. In fact, **in 2016, the percentage of Hispanic children living with married parents was 57%. This compares with 33% for Black, and 73% for White children.**

Clear associations between parental time spent with children's homework and other activities have been difficult to find. [173] However, parent participation in school life and parental involvement in home activities related to school tend to correlate with better outcomes. [82, 175] Hispanic parents appear to spend less time engaged in educational activities such as reading. Also, they tend to have lower levels of education and maternal education may be more predictive of children's development than poverty.

Type of early childhood care

The type of primary care that children under 5 years of age receive is strongly related to the level of poverty of their caregivers. The most common types of care include:

1. Center based care such as day-care centers,
5. Parents taking care of their own children at home,
6. Relatives taking care of the children at home,
7. Non-relatives such as nannies taking care of the children at home,
8. A combination of two or more of the above.

Factors rated as "very important" by parents when selecting weekly care arrangements (selected factors by race White or Hispanic)

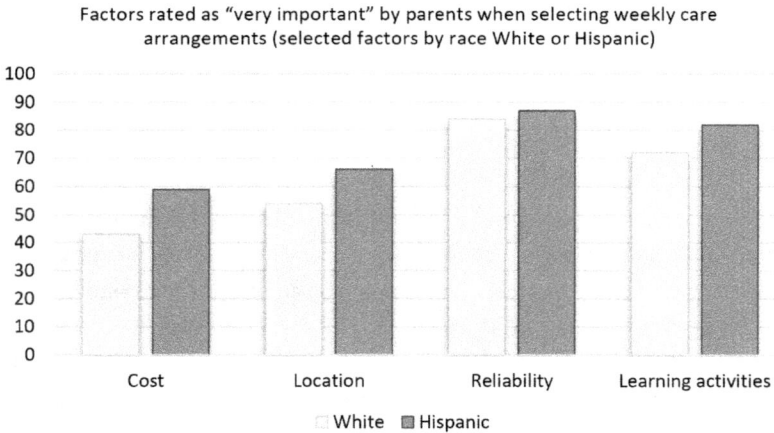

FIGURE 40. FACTORS RATED AS IMPORTANT WHEN SELECTING WEEKLY CARE ARRANGEMENTS

When asked to choose the most important factor for making care arrangements for their children, almost 6 out of 10 Hispanic parents say cost and location are "very important." Only 4 out of 10 White parents say the same. [176]

Because of the high cost, **the percentage of children who regularly receive center-based care is lower for Hispanic children than for White children**. Conversely, the percentage of children receiving parental care is higher for children from poor families and for Hispanic children compared to Whites.

Based on electronic searches of studies, expert commentaries, and policy statements addressing important aspects of early childhood development in Latino children, Salud America estimates that 42% of Hispanic children live in what they term "childcare deserts" with no or overfull early care and education centers.

Limited English Language Proficiency

Below is a list of ten key findings on this topic:

1. In the fall of 2015, about 4.9 million public school students were identified as English language learners (ELL). [87]
2. Approximately 8 out of 10 English Language Learners (ELLs) in the U.S. are Hispanic. Many of these students were born in the U.S. but grew up speaking Spanish at home.
3. One-quarter of young Latino children live in a household where adults have difficulty speaking English. [177]
4. Only 34.5% of the Hispanics born in Latin America who live in the United States say that they speak English well. 72.4% of them speak Spanish at home. [54]
5. English language proficiency is directly associated with poverty and parents not having completed high school. Children whose primary

language is not English are much more likely to live in poverty and much less likely to have parents who completed high school. English language proficiency is associated with higher educational achievement. [82, 178]

6. Hispanic students attend schools with higher concentrations of first-year teachers who often lack any qualifications to teach students with low levels of English proficiency. According to the NCES, a very small percentage of ELL teachers (2.5%) actually have a degree in ESL or bilingual education.

7. In some schools, students with limited English proficiency are placed in separate classes taught in Spanish. While this appears to be advantageous, these students end up lagging behind their peers because of their limited language proficiency improvement over time and because they are typically not exposed to high-level classes.

8. Asians and Hispanics are the most likely second-language users as well as the groups most likely to report some tutoring or coursework needed in English preparation at college entry. [179]

9. Spanish and English vocabulary in kindergarten predicts the English literacy development through eighth grade suggesting that, at least within a Spanish-speaking bilingual student population, early age oral language instruction plays a key role in literacy scores later in life. [180, 181]

10. The Office for Civil Rights (OCR) has reported on districts that do not identify students and parents whose home language is other than English, or provide sufficient instructional time for elementary school EL students, to ensure that interpreters are available when needed.

Lack of teacher and mentor support

The effort to diversify the pool of teachers has not kept up with the rapid growth of students of color, thus the racial/ethnic gap between minority students and their teachers has increased over the years.

Several studies have demonstrated that teachers influence students' motivation and thus their ability to achieve in school. and that students who feel that they are part of a community and feel well connected with their teachers and mentors tend to be more successful. [182-184] An interesting systematic review published recently describes less supportive teachers and schools as one of the factors associated with poor outcomes in science and math among disadvantaged students. [175]

In a qualitative study conducted among Hispanics who had dropped out of public schools in the city of Lawrence, MA, [185] the investigator divided the participants into two groups a) the "opportunity youth" who are neither enrolled in school nor participating in the labor market, [186] and b) the "community leaders," who are professionals over the age of 18 who graduated from a high school in Lawrence and worked with local youth. Almost 40% of the interview time with both groups was spent talking about the importance of social interactions with peers, teachers, mentors and members of the community. But interestingly, while the "opportunity youth" saw these interactions as a risk factor for poor educational attainment, the "community leaders" saw it as a positive aspect of their educational career, suggesting a perceived a correlation between positive social interactions and educational achievement. Another interesting finding was that when looking at the individual types of social interaction, the highest rated included interactions with teachers, mentors and the community. These ratings were significantly higher than interactions with family members or peers. Furthermore, study participants said that mentors were scarce in their high school experience. However, once again, participants in the opportunity youth group described their guidance counselors as useless, unwelcoming, and un-relatable while other the community leaders, remembered their counselors as going above and beyond the call of duty to assist them in entering college.

In spite of the small size and empirical design of this study, its findings are in line with publications that have suggested that even in the absence of a supportive home environment, school climate can provide sufficient support to guarantee success. For example, one study concluded that educational success is the result of a combination of peer influence and perceptions of teacher relationship, while extracurricular activities do not directly influence academic achievement. Students are more motivated when they feel a strong sense of community within their learning environment. [183, 184]

In another study of 467 dropouts aged 16 to 25 from different geographical areas in the U.S., 66% of interviewees said they would have worked harder if their teachers and parents had had higher expectations of them. Many also said that they felt insufficiently challenged by their teachers and that classes were not motivating. [182, 187]

Mentoring is one of the most important factors for career success at all stages of the educational journey. In fact, both the Liaison Committee on Medical Education and the Accreditation Council for Graduate Medical Education has deemed mentorship as a mandatory subject in medical education.

Numerous publications around the impact of mentoring on educational outcomes and the quality of medical centers are available. [102-108, 188-191] For example, a prospective, longitudinal study conducted from 2009-2016 enrolled 23 junior faculty mentees and 91 junior faculty controls from the Departments of Radiation Oncology and Anesthesia, Critical Care and Pain Management in a formal mentorship program. The mentees reported increased satisfaction in most domains related to mentoring, compared with no change in the control group. More importantly, mentees were more likely than controls to hold senior faculty positions and to be funded and/or promoted, than controls. [190]

Of note, even though there are numerous mentorship programs in place around the country, mentoring of underrepresented groups has not typically been addressed. One example of a mentoring program in medical professions that has placed special focus on those addressing the topic of diversity is The National Research Mentoring Network (NRMN). In 2012, the National Institutes of Health (NIH) Advisory Committee published a report in which they deemed the lack of diversity among biomedical and behavioral researchers as an unacceptable.

In the report, the Working Group on Diversity in the Biomedical Research Workforce (WGDBRW) identified the availability and quality of mentoring support for graduate students and newly graduated doctorates as an important variable in successfully enhancing the proportion of URM students who will ultimately obtain an independent position in a research university, medical school, or independent research institute, and successfully compete for R01 grants — one proxy for scientific independence. [192]

As a result of this recommendation, the NIH established the "Enhancing the Diversity of the NIH-Funded Workforce" program, [193] also known as the Diversity Program Consortium, to prepare individuals of underrepresented backgrounds for success and to enhance diversity in the biomedical research workforce. The program encompasses three initiatives:

a. The National Research Mentoring Network" (NRMN)
https://nrmnet.net/#undergradPopup
b. "Building Infrastructure Leading to Diversity" (BUILD) which includes 10 schools around the country: https://diversityprogramconsortium.org/pages/build and,
c. "Coordination and Evaluation Center" (CEC) based at The University of California.

Other NIH programs include the National Heart, Lung, and Blood Institute (NHLBI) Summer Institute Programs to Increase Diversity [194] and the Programs to Increase Diversity among Individuals Engaged in Hea th-related Research (PRIDE). Several publications are available that report the characteristics of the participants as well as the outcomes to date. [194-197]

Some of the programs focus on diversity among faculty, for example, the national Initiative on Gender, Culture and Leadership in Medicine-"C-Change." [94]
A study at the University of Michigan enrolled a total of 289 students including 26% Hispanic, African American and Asian. From that sample, approximately 80% grew up in mostly White neighborhoods and about 68% claimed their friends were mostly white or nearly all White. Most of them (75%) had never participated in a diversity program. After the intervention, which involved enrollment in diversity courses, the students scored higher in several tools measuring critical thinking disposition, self-confidence, social agency (e.g. how important influencing social values, helping others who are in difficulty, participating in a community action program, and helping to promote racial understanding are to them personally), the amount of interaction students have with diverse peers, and the quality of those interactions. [198]

School segregation is another complex and controversial topic that I will only briefly address here from the point of view of its potential impact on long-term outcomes related to the health professions.

A few studies have looked at the short- and long-term consequences of school segregation, but most them focus on African American students. [199, 200] The problem is that it is difficult to conclusively determine the effect of racial segregation on long-term life achievement in isolation due to the numerous confounding factors. For example, school segregation is closely related to residential segregation. [201] For more information on school segregation, I recommend reading a recent publication by investigators from UCLA Berkeley entitled: "Worsening School Segregation for Latino Children?" [202] and the references included in that article.

Hispanics are disproportionately under enrolled in Gifted and Talented programs. Some of the initiatives put in place to help high-achieving students, such as the Gifted and Talented programs, appear to lead to segregation, an observation that has created significant controversy in places like New York City where a proposal has been put forward to eliminate such programs. [203]

It's been reported that access to advanced classes is a better predictor of long-term outcomes than socio-economic factors. [204] Schools with high percentages of Hispanic attendees often lack high-level courses such as high-level math and science, which puts these students at even higher risk of low educational attainment in the long term.

While Black and Hispanic students represent 40% of the students enrolled in schools offering Gifted and Talented programs, they represent only 26% of the students enrolled in Gifted and Talented education programs and only 18% of all students receiving a qualifying score of 3 or above on an advanced placement (AP) exam.

It has been reported that the number of students attending intensely segregated schools (schools where 90% or more of students are non-White) has tripled since 1988. According to a recent publication, the chances that a Hispanic child attends a school with White classmates has decreased [202] particularly in schools with at least a 10% Hispanic enrollment and in the nation's 10 poorest districts. This does not occur uniformly across the nation, with some areas like New York showing increased probabilities of interaction between Hispanics and White students, a phenomenon known as "integration."

Some studies that have divided students into achievement quartiles in the fourth grade, suggest that at least for African Americans, sharing the class with poor achievers increases their chance to under achieve. This may be related to peer pressure and lower expectations by teachers. These hypotheses are controversial and difficult to test, but they raise an important question related to the impact of segregation on self-perception and the so-called stereotype threat, which is an important factor in achievement in other contexts as well, as discussed earlier in this book. [68, 70]

Similarly, a study conducted at Dartmouth found that when students with low GPAs began rooming with higher-scoring students, their GPAs increased. This important peer effect demonstrates the importance of the environment in school performance. [205]

In regard to medical school segregation, I only summarize some of the historical events that have shaped the current structure of medical education in the U.S. in Box 3.

BOX 3. HISTORICAL EVENTS RELATED TO MEDICAL SCHOOL SEGREGATION

The current structure of American medical schools is by enlarge a result of the "Flexner Report," published in 1910.

Abraham Flexner was a school-teacher from Louisville, KY who attended Johns Hopkins University thanks to a gift from his brother who was a pharmacist and later head of the Rockefeller Institute. He used the proceedings from selling his private school to fund his own Master's degree education at Harvard as well as his travels to Europe where he visited schools in different countries, particularly Germany, comparing European and American education in his book entitled The American College. The Carnegie Foundation had identified the need to improve health care in America by increasing the quality of medical education and elevating the standards of requirements for the degree of M.D. by all medical schools in the U.S. Another goal was to increase the income of physicians and the competition with homeopaths.

Having read Flexner's book, the head of the Carnegie Foundation invited Flexner to survey medical schools in the U.S. and Canada. Even though Flexner had never attended medical school, the Foundation believed that the problem with medical schools in the U.S. was an educational problem and thus, a professional educator would be in a better position to evaluate it and provide recommendations.

Flexner believed that the German model of Medical education was the ideal. In Germany, physicians were trained as laboratory scientists as a pre-requisite for clinical training. He collaborated with Johns Hopkins University and used it as the "gold standard" against which he compared all medical schools for his report categorizing them as (1) schools comparable to Johns Hopkins, (2) schools considered substandard but which could be improved with financial assistance, or (3) schools with quality so poor that closure was necessary.

Flexner personally visited 168 medical schools in the U.S. and Canada. He focused on the actual facilities, laboratory equipment, scientific acumen of the instructors, access hospitals, students' ability to practice more than simply observe, admissions requirements, and other factors.

This powerful report helped convert medical schools to a more scientific structure requiring the teaching of science and technology. The consequences of the Flexner report on the medical education of African Americans is well known. It led to the reduction of the seven existing African American medical schools to two, due to the report's conclusion that medical care to the African American race "should never be wholly left to African American physicians." Also well-known are the anti-Semitic statements included in the report which led to protests after its publication.

Less talked about are the consequences of Flexner's recommendations on medical education for other minorities in the U.S. This is difficult to determine because Hispanics were not counted in census until the 1970s and 80s and at least three historical events took place since the early 1960s that have influenced the participation of minorities in high education.

1. Federal agencies were required to have affirmative action plans in place in the mid '60s;
2. Title VII of the Public Health Service Act provided funding resulting in a very significant increase in the number of medical students and residents between 1970 and 1984; and
3. In the mid-2000's, the Association of American Medical Colleges recommended a 30% increase in the physician supply in response to a report by the Council on Graduate Medical Education (COGME) warning about increased needs due to the growing U.S. population, the increased number covered by health insurance plans and the aging of the baby boomers.

It is not difficult to understand why exposure to violent crime in school can contribute to low educational attainment. However, as with the other risk factors, it is difficult to attribute poor educational achievement late in life exclusively to this factor in isolation. Schools with high prevalence of criminal events tend to host a number of other risk factors.

Nevertheless, several scholars who have looked at the influence of violence in school outcomes have concluded that violent crime appears to have a direct, negative impact on student learning as measured for example by math and reading scores. [206-208]

KEY FINDINGS:

1. 5% of Hispanic students in grades 9–12 reported carrying a weapon on school property at least 1 day during the previous 30 days. This compares with 4% of White students. [209]
2. 6% of Hispanic students reported being threatened or injured with a weapon on school property, compared with 5% of White students. [209] However, this percentage decreased significantly from 2007 (8.7%).
3. Among Hispanic and Black students exposed to violent crime before the ELA test in New York City, those students attending the least safe schools and who were exposed to community violence before the test scored 0.06 standard deviations lower, which is equivalent to 40% of the test score gap between poor and non-poor students in the study population. The largest effect was seen among Hispanic students in the least safe schools who scored 0.09 standard deviations lower. The authors conclude that stronger school climates might offer a protective effect for Hispanic students. A hypothesis that may explain negative findings by other authors. [210]

4. During the school year of 2016 alone, the Office of Civil Rights received 2,450 complaints on Bullying and Harassment on the Basis of Race, Color, and National Origin and claims to have resolved 2,218 of them. [211]

Several illustrative examples are mentioned in the OCR report, including one in which a Hispanic student approached an English-speaking teacher to tell him that he had fallen and hurt his head. The teacher dismissed him because he was unable to explain the injury in English. Over an hour later the student was finally able to explain the injury to a Spanish-speaking teacher who looked for medical attention for the student.

Low school quality

Hispanic students reap the same benefits of higher-level math and science courses as do non-Hispanic White students. [212] Unfortunately, segregation among many factors has left poor and minority schools with lower-quality facilities, larger class sizes, and less effective teachers. [213]

Over half of Hispanic (60%) and Black (58%) students attended public schools in which the combined enrollment of minority students was at least 75% of the total enrollment. In contrast, only 5% of White students attended such schools.

Independent of race/ethnicity, it is important to note that only 48% of high schools in the United States offer calculus courses, only 60% offer physics and 72% offer chemistry courses. Between 10% and 25% of high schools do not offer more than one of the core courses in the typical sequence of high school math and science education—such as Algebra I and II, geometry, biology, and chemistry.

Specific to the Hispanic population:

1. As many as one quarter of high schools with the highest percentage of Black and Latino students do not offer Algebra II; and a third of these schools do not offer chemistry [211]
2. Only 33% of high schools with high Black and Hispanic student enrollment offer calculus, compared to 56% of schools with low black and Hispanic student enrollment. [211]
3. Hispanic students attend schools with higher concentrations of first-year teachers than do White students, and this is even more pronounced among English learners.

High retention rates

It is known that retention in the early school grades increases the odds that a student will drop out of school before graduating high school.

One study followed more than seven hundred Texas school children for 14 years to investigate differences in high school completion between students that are retained in Grades 1–5 versus those that are continuously promoted. The study showed that Hispanic girls are particularly susceptible to be affected in the long-term when they struggle at young age. [214]

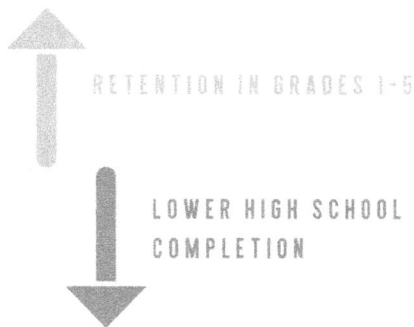

RETENTION IN GRADES 1-5

LOWER HIGH SCHOOL COMPLETION

FIGURE 41 HIGH RETENTION RATES EQUAL LOW HIGH SCHOOL COMPLETION

Unfortunately, there is no common measure of high school dropout or graduation rates at the school level and since states are allowed to use different measures, identifying which high schools have high dropout rates is difficult. The NCES **uses the term "status dropout rate" to represent the percentage of 16- through 24-year-olds who are not enrolled in school and have not earned a high school credential** (either a diploma or an equivalency credential such as a General Educational Development [GED] certificate).

The Hispanic status dropout rate has decreased from 2000 to 2016 (27.8 to 8.6%). This is encouraging, even though the rate remained higher than the Black and White rates. Importantly, the rates vary among Hispanics of different descent. For example, the high school status dropout rate was 2.4% for individuals of Peruvian descent, 6.1 for Ecuadorians and 22.9% for those of Guatemalan descent. [165]

Among the demographic characteristics associated with risk to dropout from high school are: [182]

1. Coming from a low-income family,
2. being a member of a racial or ethnic minority group,
3. being older than the average student in that grade and
4. being male.

In their paper "Locating the Dropout Crisis," [215] Robert Balfanz and Nettie Legters describe a measure that they call "promoting power," which compares the number of freshmen at a high school to the number of seniors four years later. High schools with the worst promoting power correspond to those that promote 50% or fewer freshmen to senior status on time. They go further to try and quantify the number of schools with 60% promoting power that correspond to schools in which graduating is not even the norm and which they call "Dropout Factories." They identify 2,000 such schools and conclude that they are primarily attended by minority students.

Balfanz and Legters make important conclusions related to Hispanic students:

1. Nearly 40% of Latino students versus only 11% of White students attend high schools in which graduation is *not* the norm.
2. 80% of high schools with the worst promoting power (measured as promote 50% or fewer freshmen to senior status on time) are concentrated in states with a high concentration of Hispanic students e.g. Arizona, California, Georgia, Florida, Illinois, Louisiana, Michigan, Mississippi, New Mexico, New York, North Carolina, Ohio, Pennsylvania, South Carolina, and Texas.
3. Compared to a majority White school, a majority minority high school is five times more likely to promote less than half freshmen to senior status on time. There are few exceptions of high schools which educate predominately minority students but have strong promoting power. These schools are primarily located in large metropolitan areas like New York City, Newark and Philadelphia, as well as in affluent suburban areas near New York City.
4. However, large cities including New York City, Philadelphia and others such as Los Angeles and Chicago, contain one-third of the schools with the lowest promoting power. In cities with high concentration of high schools that have a low promoting power, there is no option for many students than to attend one of these schools.
5. The strongest correlate to high schools with low promoting power is poverty.

One important aspect associated with dropouts at the college level is the "sense of belonging." Many students coming from public schools feel alienated in college, [216] especially if they manage to access top schools with environments that are unfamiliar. [140] Also, Hispanics are more likely to attend community colleges, which some researchers have found often discourage further advancement among minority students, a phenomenon known as the "cooling out hypothesis" which has recently been revisited and revised in an interesting study by K. Broton which takes financial aid into account. [217]

According to the Center for Labor Market Studies, high school dropouts earn $9,200 less per year on average than those who graduate and over the course of their lifetimes, they will earn an average of $375,000 less than high school graduates, and $1 million less than college graduates.

Key takeaways from chapter 4

1

The main risk factors for low educational attainment are poverty, limited English proficiency and low school quality.

2

Establishing a direct relationship between a child's early environment and their achievement later in life is difficult because multiple factors play a role. Exposure to multiple risk factors in combination has a cumulative effect on long-term outcomes.

3

Hispanic infants and children are less likely than children from other races to receive center-based care. 42% of Hispanic children live in areas with no or overfull early child-care and education centers. However, Hispanic children may have an advantage when it comes to living arrangements because they often live in stable, two-parent households with parents who are steadily employed. In 2016, the percentage of Hispanic children living with married parents was 57%. This compares with 33% for Blacks, and 73% for White children.

4

Segregation of low income and minority students begins early in life. The number of students attending intensely segregated schools (schools where 90% or more of students are non-White) has tripled since 1988.

5

The Hispanic status dropout rate has decreased between 2000 and 2016 (27.8% to 8.6%).

6

Mentoring is one of the most important factors for career success at all stages of the educational journey. The presence of supportive teachers and schools is one of the factors associated with better outcomes throughout the educational journey.

Online resources for chapter 4

IF YOU ARE INTERESTED IN:	GO TO:
Family and Household Composition, Family Formation and Stability, Relationship Dynamics, Parenting	Hispanic Research Center: https://www.hispanicresearchcenter.org/research-resources/data-tool-measuring-hispanic-families-and-households/
Childcare assistance for low-income families.	The Child Care and Development Block Grant (CCDBG) is the largest federal funding source to help states provide child care assistance to low-income families. [218]
Information on school violence	Two key sources of are the Youth Risk Behavior Survey (YRBS), conducted by the Youth Risk Behavior Surveillance System (YRBSS) at the Centers for Disease Control and Prevention https://www.cdc.gov/healthyyouth/data/yrbs/index.htm and the School Crime Supplement (SCS) to the National Crime Victimization Survey. https://safesupportivelearning.ed.gov/survey/school-crime-supplement-scs-national-crime-victimization-survey-ncvs

| Reporting and data collection on school violence and civil rights | Department of Education's Office for Civil Rights (OCR) Ongoing online effort of the DOE to make data collection and sharing transparent and available to the public. |

WHY DO WE NEED MORE HISPANIC DOCTORS?

When you think of health disparities, you usually think of problems with unequal access to health care, or the impact of things like poverty and unsafe neighborhoods. But there are disparities in the health care children receive, even after they're in our hospitals."
— Casey Lion, MD, MPH, Pediatrician, Seattle Children's, and Researcher, Center for Child Health, Behavior and Development

CHAPTER FIVE

HISPANIC HEALTH BY THE NUMBERS

"Of all the forms of inequality, injustice in health care is the most shocking and inhumane."
– Martin Luther King

In previous chapters, I have described the difficulties quantifying the underrepresentation of Hispanics in Medicine in the U.S. In this section I go beyond the numbers to describe why more Hispanic physicians are needed.

Because of all the reasons described so far, estimation of the shortage of Hispanic physicians in the U.S. is difficult. **However, the real question that no model takes into account is how much the health status of the Hispanic population could improve by ensuring that the diversity in healthcare professions matches the country's racial and ethnic diversity. Data on this topic is severely lacking.[219] However, most available data and the testimonies from patients and healthcare providers suggest that racial, ethnic, linguistic and culturally competent health care correlates with better access to care and quality of care among disadvantaged. It is easier for people to receive care if their doctors speak their language or if they are at least aware of the cultural aspects related to their determinants of health.**

Diversity in the healthcare workforce is a moral and public policy imperative and the reasons for increased diversity listed below, which have been proposed by many others, do not indicate that minority physicians are obligated to care for underserved populations, or that White physicians or physicians of other races cannot care for those populations. Instead, the focus is on improved, more culturally and linguistically competent care.

I first review the available information on cultural and linguistic competence in health care and then go on to describe the current health status of the Hispanic population in the U.S. In the next chapter, I present examples of culturally and linguistically competent programs that have used in an attempt to improve major determinants of health.

ANA MARIA'S SISTER KEEPS MISSING HER TREATMENT BECAUSE HER PARENTS CANNOT AFFORD IT

"I'm sorry for being late Mrs. Martinez," Ana Maria says to her school counselor. "My sister is at the hospital and I needed to help. As you know, my parents don't speak English and someone needed to explain the doctor what happened with my sister after her insulin injection last night.

Ana Maria felt conflicted. "I kept asking myself, how can my parents help with my college education when they can't even afford a life-saving treatment for my sister!"

Even though Hispanics experience lower rates of mortality than people from other races/ethnicities, there is a lot of heterogeneity among Hispanic subgroups. For example, Hispanics, particularly Mexican Americans and Puerto Ricans suffer disproportionately from diabetes. [220-222] In addition, Hispanics have lower levels of health insurance and access to health care. In this chapter, we will look at the data on the health status of the Hispanic population in the U.S.

Health is multidimensional

In the same way as the definition of a Hispanic/Latino is narrow and does not take into account the many dimensions of Hispanic identity, the definition of health is also narrow, and does not take into account the multiple dimensions that matter to most people, which include physical, mental, and social aspects, collectively known as quality of life.

Many of these aspects refer to people's own perceptions of well-being that are difficult to measure, which is why scientists and epidemiologists often focus on objective outcomes such as rates of disease (morbidity) and death (mortality) as measures of the overall health status of a population.

In the same way as we arrived at a new definition of race and racial identity, there is a new definition of health, beyond the physical aspects. According to this definition, a person's health is determined by complex interactions between genetics, environmental, social and economic factors and individual behaviors such as dietary choices.

All these factors are collectively known as **determinants of health** [223] and are defined as "a range of personal, social, economic and environmental factors that influence the health status of individuals and populations."

The WHO included quality of life as part of their definition of health decades ago.

"Health is a state of complete physical, mental, and social well-being—not merely the absence of disease, or infirmity."
−World Health Organization, 1948

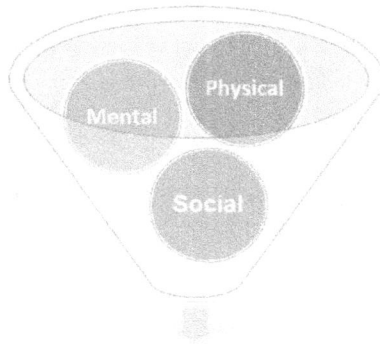

Quality of life

FIGURE 42. QUALITY OF LIFE

As a result, several measures of quality of life are now routinely used when evaluating the effect of different interventions. Two examples of questions asked to evaluate people's quality of life are: [224]

- Would you say that in general your health is excellent, very good, good, fair, or poor?
- Thinking about your mental health, which includes stress, depression, and problems with emotions, for how many days during the past 30 days was your mental health not good?

Individuals cannot control all determinants of health. Thus, several organizations have set out to improve the health status of the population over time by identifying quantifiable **health status indicators** related to key determinants of health, to monitor progress over time in response to policy changes and other initiatives. One such organization in the U.S. is the Office of disease prevention and promotion, which funds a program called "Healthy People Initiative." The goal of the Healthy People Initiative is to improve the health status of the population over time and to create a society in which everyone has a chance to live a long, healthy life. The Healthy People Initiative has included quality of life improvement as a central public health goal.

Every decade, the Healthy People Initiative develops a new set of science-based, 10-year national objectives with the goal of improving the health of all Americans. The original list of 18 health status indicators has been revised over time. There is a subset of "**leading health indicators**" which represent top priority health issues and challenges.

In the current iteration of the Healthy People Initiative (Healthy People 2020), the list of leading health indicators is organized in 12 topics:
1. Access to Health Services
2. Clinical Preventive Services
3. Environmental Quality
4. Injury and Violence
5. Maternal, Infant, and Child Health
6. Mental Health
7. Nutrition, Physical Activity, and Obesity
8. Oral Health
9. Reproductive and Sexual Health
10. Social Determinants
11. Substance Abuse
12. Tobacco use

A detailed discussion of determinants of health, particularly social determinants, is beyond the scope of this book and more information can be found at the Healthy People Initiative website: https://www.healthypeople.gov/.

Once one of the factors is affected, all others can be influenced as well (Figure 43). For example, a low-income population spends less on education and housing, and has lower levels of insurance and educational attainment, which is related to increased exposure to violence, poor environmental quality, mental health issues and higher rates of substance abuse. Individuals who secure stable employment are more likely to live in neighborhoods with higher quality schools and lower rates of violence, crime and lower prevalence of preventable diseases. Low socioeconomic status is associated with an increased risk for many diseases, including cardiovascular disease, arthritis, diabetes, chronic respiratory diseases, and cervical cancer, as well as mental conditions.

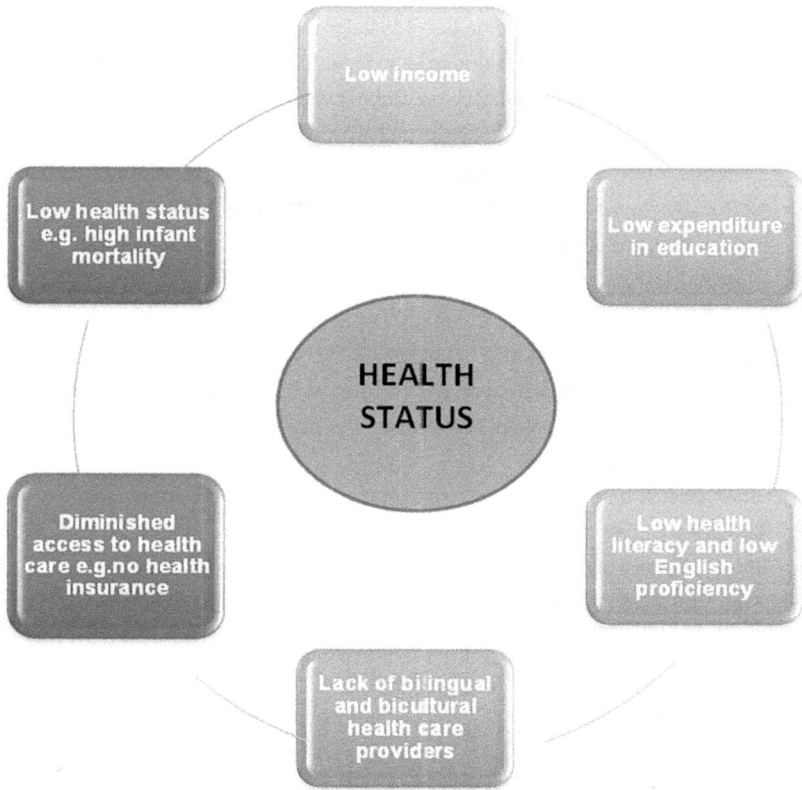

FIGURE 43. DETERMINANTS OF HEALTH. PERSONAL, SOCIAL, ECONOMIC AND ENVIRONMENTAL FACTORS INTERACT WITH EACH OTHER TO CONTRIBUTE TO THE HEALTH OF AN INDIVIDUAL OR A POPULATION

Some of the social determinants of health relevant to the Hispanic population due to known disparities based on race and ethnicity are:

- Socioeconomic conditions like concentrated poverty and residential segregation
- Social norms and attitudes, such as discrimination
- Social aspects such as "familism" which constitutes one of the key Latino values, heavily relied upon when dealing with health problems and related to the fact that family takes precedence when making healthcare decisions [225]
- Social support and social interactions
- Immigration status

- Unequal distribution of income and education; unequal access to education
- Worse access to health care due to lack of availability, high cost, lack of insurance coverage, limited transportation, language barriers and inconvenient appointment times
- Lack of familiarity with the healthcare system
- Lack of bilingual and bicultural healthcare providers to effectively communicate information about health also results in decreased access to health care
- Health literacy

This book is about the importance of increasing the number and cultural competence of healthcare providers as a mechanism to improve specific health status indicators. For that reason, I have structured this section as follows:

1. Brief discussion on the overall health status of the Hispanic population and the so-called "Hispanic paradox"
2. Brief summary of data on access to health services among Hispanics
3. Status of selected health indicators relevant to the Hispanic population along with examples of the application of bilingual and bicultural interventions that have already been shown to improve outcomes related to these indicators. [226]

The Hispanic/Latino paradox

So far in this chapter, we have talked about the fact that mortality rates alone do not accurately represent the health status of a population. We have also talked about the fact that all determinants of health are interdependent, and about the fact that quantifying the health of a population using a single measure is not ideal. For that reason, when one quantifies the health of the Hispanic population by using only mortality rates, the results are unexpected. This is what epidemiologists have called the "Hispanic paradox."

Hispanics in the U.S. have lower mortality rates than non-Hispanic Whites and non-Hispanic Blacks. This is in spite of the fact that almost all other social determinants of health are worse for Hispanics than for other races/ethnicities.

Apart from total number of deaths, another measure used is known as "avoidable mortality" and represents the number of deaths from certain causes that should not occur in the presence of timely and effective health care. This is a good measure of deaths due to preventable, treatable factors. [227] According to data from the National Vital Statistics System (NVSS), the rate of avoidable mortality between 2016 and 2017 was 66.7 per 100,000 for Hispanics, 78.5 per 100,000 for Whites and 154.9 per 100,000 for Blacks. Once again, by this measure, Hispanics fare much better than Whites and Blacks.

There are several aspects to consider when thinking about the Hispanic paradox. Like many other population-level statistic, it lumps all people into the same category without taking into account that mortality rates vary among genders, age groups, geographical regions, country of origin, occupation, among many other factors. For example, data shows that Hispanic workers are more likely to perform high-risk jobs in construction, domestic maintenance and repair services, manufacturing, and household services, as compared to Whites (59% versus 38.1%), and this increases the rate of mortality among that group of Hispanics due to occupational hazards. This is particularly true for seasonal farm workers who are exposed to pesticides, heat, skin diseases and physical injuries. [228-231] However, these increased rates are diluted when considering the overall population, and in some cases, migrants who are seasonal workers are not counted in the statistics because of their immigration status and the fact that they do not participate in the census or other health surveys.

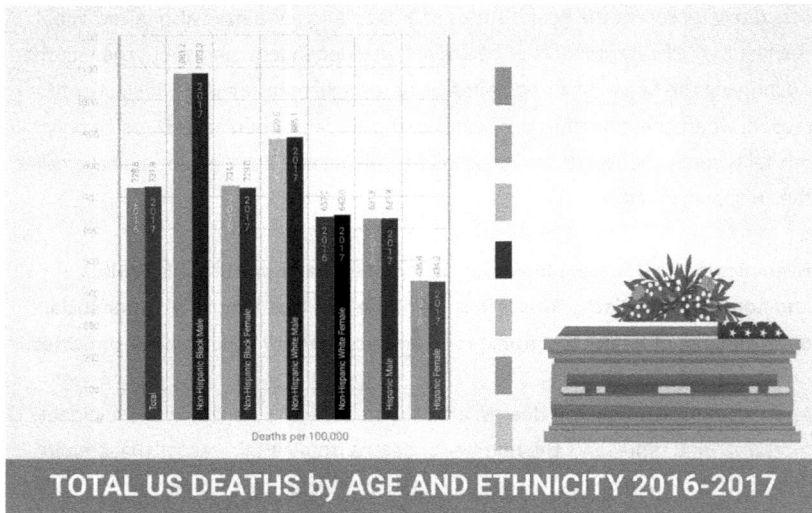

TOTAL US DEATHS by AGE AND ETHNICITY 2016-2017

FIGURE 44. TOTAL U.S. DEATHS BY AGE AND ETHNICITY

Other examples include obesity and type 2 diabetes, which occur more frequently among certain subgroups of Hispanics, such as Mexican-Americans, resulting in increased mortality due to these causes within this group, as well as hypertension which is present in more than 30% of Dominican men, but only 15% of South American women. Once again, these differences get lost when the entire Hispanic population is considered as a whole. Importantly, it has been predicted that type 2 diabetes will increase, making the differences in mortality between Hispanics and Whites fade over time. [232]

One hypothesis proposed to explain the Hispanic paradox is that lower smoking rates among Hispanics drive their decreased mortality. Another observation is that Hispanics are overall a younger population (~15 years younger) than Whites. Yet, another theory is that recent migrants are healthier than non-Hispanic Whites skewing the mortality rates down for the entire Hispanic population. [233] Supporters of this latter theory claim that Hispanic health is better among those who recently migrated to the U.S. from other countries, even compared to U.S.-born Hispanics. [234] Either it is the healthiest individuals that immigrate to the U.S., that health behaviors outside of the U.S. are more favorable, or that sick individuals return to their countries of origin.

However, recent studies do not support this hypothesis and suggest that **even though Hispanics live longer lives, their lives are harder due to socioeconomic hardship, stress and health risks**. [235] This brings us back to the discussion around quality of life and the fact that comparisons in hard outcomes such as death fail to take into account aspects of health that really matter to people.

This is relevant to our discussion because as mentioned throughout the book, our goal should be to improve people's quality of life and ensure that everyone, regardless of their race or socioeconomic status receives appropriate, timely, culturally and linguistically competent health care.

The Hispanic Community Health Study/Study of Latinos (HCHS/SOL) is a large multicenter study that includes more than 16,000 Hispanics and collects extensive information on health outcomes and genetics among Latinos in four U.S. metropolitan areas. This study has generated a large number of publications and will most certainly continue to shed light on many of the questions around the health of the Hispanic population in the U.S.

The Latina paradox

Infants born to Hispanic mothers have been shown to be less likely to experience low birth weight (LBW: infants weighing less than 2500 grams or 5 pounds, 8 ounces at birth) and infant mortality, compared with infants of White women. This is known as the "Latina paradox."

The percentage of LBW infants born to Hispanic mothers has increased year after year since 2010 from 6.9 to 7.4%, while the rate for infants born to non-Hispanic White mothers has decreased slightly during the same period of time from 7.3 to 7.0%.

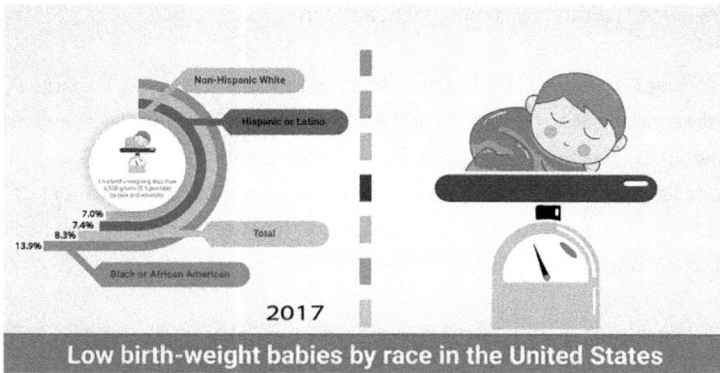

FIGURE 45. LOW BIRTH-WEIGHT BABIES BY RACE IN THE UNITED STATES

There are differences among Hispanic subgroups. In general, U.S.-born Hispanic women have a similar or greater risk of adverse outcomes compared with Whites and foreign-born Hispanic women. Foreign-born Hispanic women had a consistently lower risk for preterm birth, LBW and small-for-gestational-age births than U.S.-born Latinas. [236] These differences may explain the increased percentage of LBW infants born to Hispanic women over time. Alternatively, as some investigators have proposed, there was no Latina paradox to begin with [237] and, at least in California, Latinas have worse birth outcomes than White women, which is consistent with their socioeconomic disadvantages.

Another factor to take into account is variability according to country of origin. For example, Puerto Ricans have a low birth weight rate twice as high as that of Whites, and suffer disproportionately from infant mortality.

In terms of infant mortality, defined as the death of an infant before his or her first birthday, the rate of infant deaths per 1,000 live births in 2017 was 5.0 for White, 5.0 for Hispanic and 11.0 for Blacks. As with other outcomes, there are clear differences among discrete subgroups. [238-240] For instance, Hispanic Black mothers experience higher odds of infant mortality than Hispanic Whites, regardless of their sociodemographic characteristics. [241]

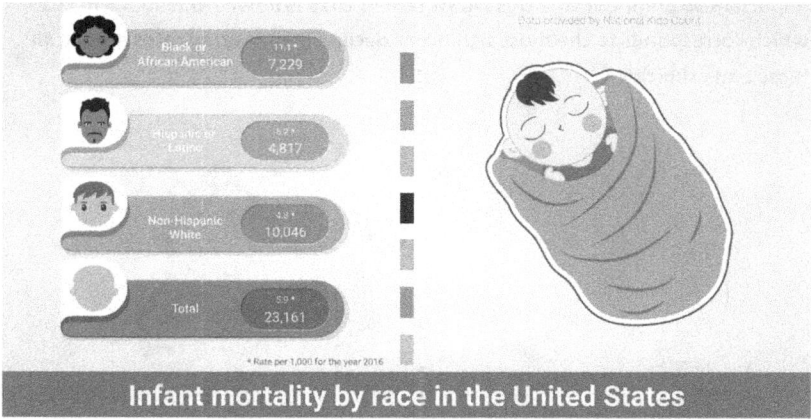

FIGURE 46. INFANT MORTALITY BY RACE AND ETHNICITY IN THE UNITED STATES

Access to Health Services

Even though the number of Hispanics who are uninsured has decreased significantly since 2010, Hispanics remain the highest uninsured minority in the United States.

According to a report from the National Center for Health Statistics based on a sample of 19,510 individuals, during the first 3 months of 2018, 24.2% of Hispanics, 14.1% of non-Hispanic Blacks, 8.9% of non-Hispanic Whites, and 6.4% Asian Whites between the ages of 18 and 64 had no health insurance. [242] **However, it is important to point out that this 24.3% rate in 2018 is down from 40.6% in 2013 which corresponds to the most significant decline in uninsured rates among all races and ethnicities.**

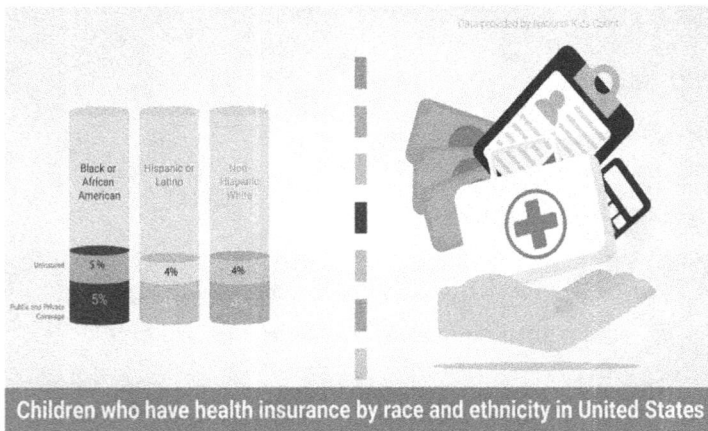

Children who have health insurance by race and ethnicity in United States

FIGURE 47. HEALTH INSURANCE STATUS BY RACE AND ETHNICITY IN THE UNITED STATES

Many Hispanics are not enrolled in public health programs because they are simply not aware of them or because of language barriers. It has been reported that as many as 70% of uninsured Latino children are eligible for Medicaid or CHIP coverage. Even those who earn above the poverty level are less likely to be insured and have lower levels of insurance coverage through their employers. Importantly, the health insurance rate is significantly higher among those with an advanced degree, compared with those without a high school education.

Clinical Preventive Services

The Healthy People Initiative defines clinical preventive services as those aimed at preventing and detecting illnesses and diseases in their earlier, more treatable stages, significantly reducing the risk of illness, disability, early death, and high medical care costs. Some examples include cancer screening and blood pressure control.

In this section I provide a brief summary of the statistical data around selected clinical preventive services corresponding to the leading causes of death among Hispanics i.e. heart disease, cancer and diabetes. In the next chapter I will provide numerous examples of initiatives that have aimed at improving health indicators among Hispanics in the U.S., by applying culturally and linguistically appropriate education.

Leading causes of death among Hispanic females by age group, 2017

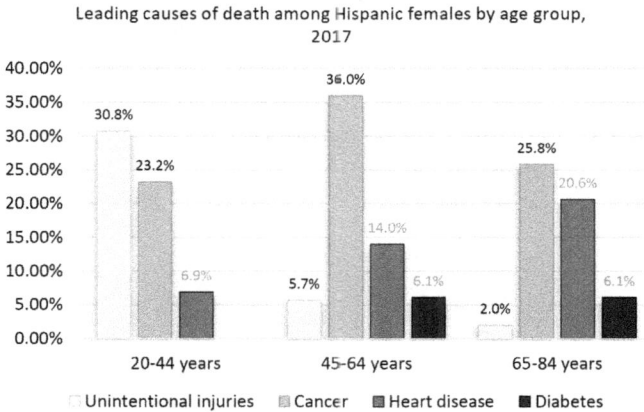

FIGURE 48. LEADING CAUSES OF DEATH AMONG HISPANIC FEMALES, 2017 (SEE NOTES ON RANKING METHODOLOGY IN THE REPORT[243])

The 2008 National Healthcare Disparities report stated that Hispanics receive less advice on exercise and heart attack-related care than White patients, in spite of the fact that:

1. Heart disease is the leading cause of death among Hispanics older than 84, and the second leading cause of death among those between the ages of 45 and 84, both male and female. [243]
2. Hispanics have higher rates of obesity overall than non-Hispanic Whites, although there are disparities among subgroups and genders, with Hispanic women at higher risk of obesity than men and U.S.-born Hispanics at higher risk than foreign-born Hispanics. [244, 245]
3. Hispanics, particularly Mexican Americans and Puerto Ricans suffer disproportionately from diabetes. [220-222]
4. Hispanic children have a 50% chance of developing diabetes in his/her lifetime due to main risk factors like obesity and lack of physical activity.

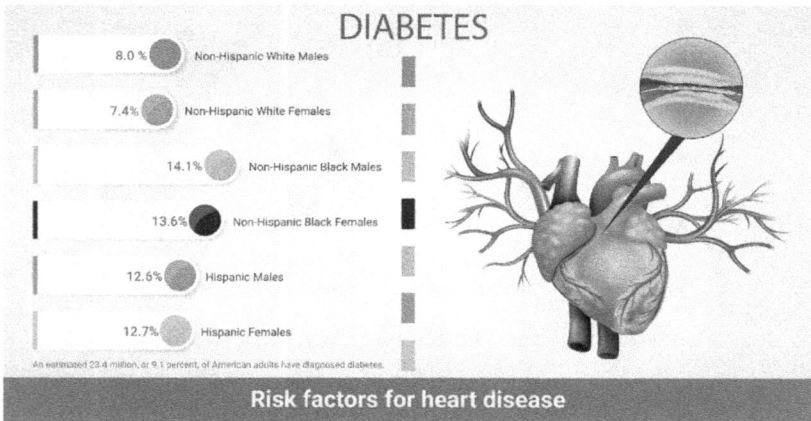

FIGURE 49. PREVALENCE OF DIABETES BY RACE AND ETHNICITY

According to the measure of health disparities conducted by the Healthy People Initiative, when comparing the proportion of persons with diagnosed diabetes, it is estimated that Mexican Americans have a 2.651 times higher rate than White, non-Hispanics. In some of the Texas-Mexico border counties, up to 50% of Mexican Americans older than 35 are diagnosed with Type 2 diabetes. [246] The mechanism behind this high prevalence of diabetes among Mexican Americans appears to be related to genetic predisposition, more than to obesity. [247]

Cancer

Cancer is the leading cause of death among both female and male Hispanics between the ages of 45 and 84. [243, 248] More than 22,000 Hispanic men and more than 20,000 Hispanic women were expected to die from cancer in 2018, with lung cancer being the main cause of death among men, and breast cancer being the main cause of death among women. [248]

However, Hispanics have lower mortality due to cancer than Whites and Blacks.

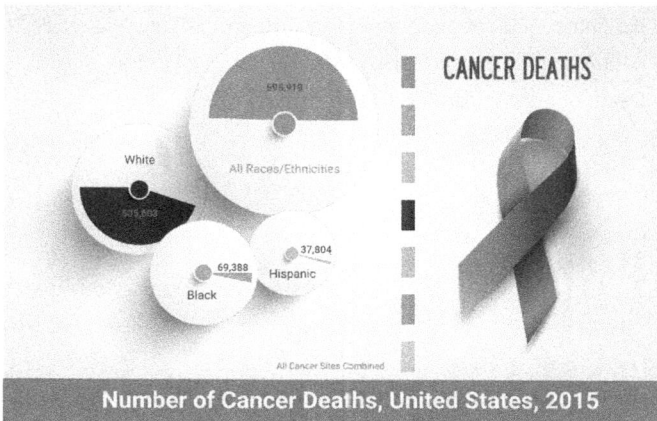

FIGURE 50. NUMBER OF CANCER DEATHS, U.S. 2015

Even though the incidence of breast cancer is lower among Hispanic females, it is the most common type of cancer among them. [243] The 5-year survival rates are lower among Hispanics when compared to non-Hispanic Whites and their mortality rates have not gone down as much as the rates among non-Hispanic Whites. [249] Some of the factors associated with these disparities are:

1. Metastatic breast cancer occurs at younger ages among Latinas and survival rates are lower. [250]

2. Hispanic females undergo genetic testing with lower frequency and show lower rates of cancer risk management practices, even among those who already carry a pathogenic BRCA mutation. [251]

3. Relevant for this book, **language barriers affect the likelihood of Hispanic women to undergo preventive and genetic testing**. One study found that discussion about genetic testing with a provider is nearly 2 times less likely among Spanish-speaking Hispanic women compared with non-Hispanic White women. [251]

4. 4. Hispanic women have a higher risk for estrogen- and progesterone-negative tumors, which are more difficult to treat and are associated with lower survival rates. [252]

5. 5. Hispanic women are more likely to identify a family member as the final treatment decision-maker. Furthermore, the less acculturated, the more likely they are to say that their family members make treatment decisions. [253]

Reproductive and sexual health

According to the CDC, adult and adolescent Hispanics made up 26% (9,889) of the 38,739 new HIV diagnoses in the United States. At the end of 2016, it is estimated that as many as 254,600 Hispanics had HIV and there were 2,863 deaths among Hispanics/Latinos with diagnosed HIV.

Many Hispanics do not use prevention services or get tested, for fear of disclosing their immigration status. Among Hispanic men, the most frequent type of transmission is male-to-male sexual contact and injection drug use.

Only 16.8% of Hispanic high school students who are sexually active report having used effective hormonal birth control the last time they had sex. This compares with 37.4% of White and 22.5% of Black students. [209] Similarly, only approximately half of Hispanic high school students report having used a condom, but there are no significant differences among races in the use of condoms. When looking at dual methods, such as hormonal birth control along with condom use, the Hispanic youth group fares the worst, with only 4% reporting to have used dual methods, compared to 11.6% of Whites.

The **Let's Stop HIV Together** campaign, also available in Spanish (Detengamos Juntos el VIH), provides culturally and linguistically appropriate messages about HIV testing, prevention, and treatment.

The **Tú No Me Conoces** social marketing campaign was an 8-week campaign that included Spanish-language radio, print media, a Web site, and a toll-free HIV-testing referral hotline to support HIV risk awareness among Hispanics living in the U.S.-Mexico border. This intervention resulted in increased HIV testing in participating clinics with almost a third of testers specifically mentioning the campaign as the reason for the visit. [254]

BOX 4. TOTAL FERTILITY RATE, BIRTHRATES AND CONTRACEPTION AMONG HISPANICS IN THE U.S.

The total fertility rate (TFR) is defined as the expected number of births that a group of 1,000 women would have in their lifetimes according to the current age-specific birth rates for the United States. In 2017 the TFR was of 1,765.5 and thus 16% below what is considered the level for a population to replace itself (2,100.0). However, among Hispanic women, 29 states had TFRs above 2,100.0. [255]

However, when looking at the data over time, the birthrate among Hispanic women fell by 31% from 2006 to 2017, compared to 5% for White women and 11% for Black women. Contributing factors may include increases in average levels of education, relatively high costs of living, and perhaps more importantly changing attitudes about childbearing. In addition, foreign-born Hispanic women generally have higher fertility than U.S.-born Hispanic women. [256]

Over the past decade, the U.S. Hispanic population has become more likely to be born in the United States. (In 2006, 54.9% of the adult Hispanic population was foreign born, compared to 47.9% in 2015.) If Hispanic fertility continues to decline, it may push the total fertility rate in the United States—already at 1.77 children per woman—further below replacement level (a total fertility rate of 2.1 children per woman, on average). [257] Yet, the significance of this on the demand for Hispanic physicians is unknown and difficult to model.

In terms of contraception, the percentage of non-Hispanic White women currently using contraception was not different from the percentage for Hispanic women (67.0% vs 64.0%), according to the most recent report NHCS report on contraceptive status among women aged 15–49. [258]

Mental Health

Minorities have, in general, equal or better mental health than White Americans, yet they suffer from disparities in mental health care.

Racial and ethnic minority patients underutilize mental health services (U.S. Surgeon General, 2001). Hispanics with mental health conditions are less likely than Whites to receive treatment. If treated, they are likely to see primary care physicians, as opposed to mental health specialists.

Using data from the National Latino and Asian American Study, Alegria and colleagues reported a lifetime psychiatric disorder prevalence estimate of 28.1% for men and 30.2% for women. [259] However, Hispanics and Blacks report lower risk of having a psychiatric disorder as compared with their White counterparts. [260, 261] In spite of the higher rates of poverty among minority individuals as compared with Whites in the U.S, all subgroups of minorities (with the exception of Puerto Ricans) reported lower rates of lifetime mental disorders than do White Americans. [262] As a matter of fact, other studies have also shown that the lowest risk for psychiatric disorders among minorities was more pronounced at lower levels of education. [261]

The suicide rate among Hispanics in 2017 was 6.9 per 100,000 population, compared with 17.8 among Whites. The percentage of adolescents (ages 12-17) with a major depressive episode in the past 12 months is the same among Hispanics and Whites at 15.1%. That percentage among adults (18+) is lower among Hispanics 6.2% than Whites 7.5%.

Even though the prevalence rates of psychiatric disorders are lower among Hispanics, it's been suggested that those who become ill tend to have more persistent and more severe disease [263, 264] and some subgroups receive inadequate care. For instance, the percentage of children (4–17 years) with mental health problems receiving treatment is lower among Hispanics (63.8%) than Whites (74.4%).

Key takeaways from chapter 5

1

In the same way as we arrived at a new definition of race and racial identity, there is a new definition of health that goes beyond the physical aspects to include physical, mental, and social aspects, collectively known as quality of life. According to this definition, a person's health is determined by complex interactions between genetics, environmental, social and economic factors, and individual behaviors such as dietary choices, collectively known as determinants of health.

2

When one quantifies the health of the Hispanic population by using only mortality rates, not taking into account quality of life, the results are unexpected. This is what epidemiologists have called the "Hispanic paradox." Hispanics in the U.S. have lower mortality rates than non-Hispanic Whites and non-Hispanic Blacks. This is in spite of the fact that almost all other social determinants of health are worse for Hispanics than for other races/ethnicities.

3

Adult and adolescent Hispanics made up almost one third of the new HIV diagnoses in the United States.

4

When quality of life is taken into account, recent studies suggest that even though Hispanics live longer, their lives are harder due to socioeconomic hardship, stress and health risks.

5

Infants born to Hispanic mothers have been shown to be less likely to experience low birth weight and infant mortality, compared with infants of White women. This is known as the "Latina paradox."

6

The most common causes of death among Hispanics are heart disease, cancer and diabetes. Hispanics have higher rates of diabetes and obesity than non-Hispanic Whites, although the prevalence varies across different groups.

7

Even though the prevalence rates of psychiatric disorders are lower among Hispanics, those who become ill tend to have more persistent and more severe disease, and some subgroups receive inadequate care.

Online resources for chapter 5

Salud América
https://salud-america.org/

The Center for Latino Adolescent and
Family Health (CLAFH)
http://clafh.org/about/
https://bhw.hrsa.gov/
loansscholarships/nhsc

America's health rankings
https://www.americashealthrankings.
org/about/methodology/introduction

Inter-university Consortium for
Political and Social Research
ICPSR is an international
consortium of more than 750
academic institutions and research
organizations, that maintains an
archive with data on social and
behavioral fields ranging from
education to substance abuse and
other fields. It is housed by University
of Michigan and open for public use.

Child Health data Stats

Child Stats
https://www.childstats.gov/
americaschildren/health2.asp

Multimedia	https://corazonfilm.com/ Montefiore's Hospital movie on organ transplantation is an excellent example of the use of media to educate around health needs.
The National Health Interview Survey (NHIS)	https://www.cdc.gov/nchs/nhis/index.htm This survey has monitored the health of the nation since 1957 and it includes data from 75,000 a 100,000 people.
Minority Health	U.S. Department of Health & Human Services https://www.minorityhealth.hhs.gov/
Insurance programs for Hispanics	https://www.cuidadodesalud.gov/es/

CHAPTER SIX

HISPANIC HEALTH BEYOND THE NUMBERS

Why do we need more Hispanic doctors in the U.S.?

"Diversity in Health Care is not about fair representation,
it's about saving lives"
– Commissioner George Strait, Associate Vice Chancellor for Public
Affairs, University of California, Berkeley

ANA MARIA HELPS WITH HER FAMILY'S INTERACTION WITH THE DOCTOR

"I'm sorry for being late Mrs. Martinez," Ana Maria says to her school counselor. "My sister is at the hospital and I needed to help. As you know, my parents don't speak English and someone needed to explain to the doctor what happened with my sister after her insulin injection last night."

Nothing has been the same for Ana Maria since this experience. The fact that her sister could have died because her parents could not explain the situation to the emergency room doctor helped her to understand how much Spanish-speaking doctors could help families like hers

"I used to feel demoralized," she says, "but this experience motivated me! I knew that I wanted to be a doctor to help people like my sister, but I after this experience, I realized that it's even bigger than that! I can't imagine how many families have the same experience."

What is cultural competence?

In simple words, a culturally competent professional provides information and services in the language and educational and cultural context that is most appropriate for the individuals he or she serves.

The Centers for Medicare & Medicaid Services define cultural and linguistic competence as the ability of healthcare providers and healthcare organizations to understand and respond effectively to the cultural and linguistic needs brought by the patient to the healthcare encounter.

The AAMC states **"When healthcare providers have life experience that more closely matches the experiences of their patients, patients tend to be more satisfied with their care and to adhere to medical advice. This effect has been seen in studies addressing racial, ethnic, and sexual minority communities when the demographics of healthcare providers reflect those of underserved populations."** [219]

Cultural competence acknowledges variations in customs, traditions, values, beliefs, and communication styles and takes them into account when assessing and treating individuals. "Culture" refers to integrated patterns of human behavior that include the language, thoughts, actions, customs, beliefs, and institutions of racial, ethnic, social, or religious groups. "Competence" implies having the capacity to function effectively as an individual or an organization within the context of the cultural beliefs, practices, and needs presented by patients and their communities."

Culture has a dramatic impact on overall health. [265] Importantly, even though I am not addressing religious and spiritual health practices collectively known as "ethnomedicine," this is another important aspect of the Hispanic culture that is highly prevalent and difficult to educate practitioners about due to its diversity and heterogeneity. [266]

What is linguistic competence?

The Centers for Medicare & Medicaid Services (CMS) defines linguistic competence as follows: "Providing readily available, culturally appropriate oral and written language services to limited English proficiency (LEP) members through such means as bilingual/bicultural staff, trained medical interpreters, and qualified translators."

Effective communication is always important, but it can mean the difference between life and death in certain circumstances related to life-threatening conditions such as urgent care, cancer diagnosis and treatment, and chronic disease management. [267] Effective communication is key not only during the conversation between patient and physician (clinical encounter), but also during other activities such as conversations with pharmacists, nurses, hospital registration staff, post-surgical environment, etc.

Linguistic competence is the linguistic knowledge possessed by native speakers of a language. However, effective communication is not only about language proficiency but about the ability to appreciate the culture relative to the spoken language. [268] Interpreters help, but collaborative work is needed to optimize the interactions between healthcare providers and interpreters for the benefit of the patients. [269]

Among the reasons why the lack of cultural and linguistic competence in the healthcare workforce leads to worse outcomes are:
1. Low levels of health literacy
2. Unsuccessful communication to patients about treatment options including the need for surgical procedures
3. Patient preference to only see racially concordant physicians
4. Healthcare provider explicit or implicit bias and racial variations in the use of treatments and procedures
5. Low participation in research

Health literacy

Cultural and linguistic competence is particularly relevant when communicating health related information to a population with low health literacy.

Health literacy is defined by the Institute of Medicine as **"the degree to which individuals can obtain, process, and understand the basic health information and services they need to make appropriate health decisions."**

Health literacy allows patients to understand their conditions and the treatments that will improve their overall wellbeing.

It has been reported that Hispanic adults have the lowest average health literacy score compared to adults in other racial and ethnic groups. [270-272] Other reports show that nearly 2 in 5 Hispanics have communication problems with their doctor. [135, 273]

According to data from the Robert Wood Johnson Foundation, one in five Spanish-speaking U.S. residents delayed or refused needed medical care because of language barriers.

41% of Hispanic adults have a level of literacy that is considered below basic. This compares with 9% of Whites and 14% of Blacks. 24% of Hispanics had a basic level of health literacy, compared to 19% of Whites and 33% of Blacks.

Below basic health literacy corresponds to the ability to complete tasks such as circling the date of a medical appointment on a hospital appointment slip, or understanding what it is permissible to drink before a medical test, based on a set of short instructions.

Basic health literacy corresponds to a person's ability to complete tasks such as giving two reasons a person with no symptoms of a specific disease should be tested for the disease based on information in a clearly written pamphlet.

More Hispanics have "below basic" health literacy than individuals of other races

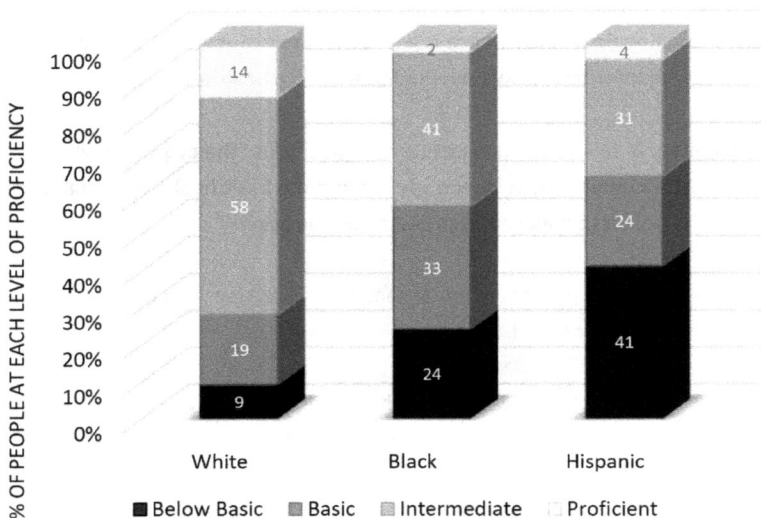

% OF PEOPLE AT EACH LEVEL OF PROFICIENCY

	White	Black	Hispanic
Proficient	14	2	4
Intermediate	58	41	31
Basic	19	33	24
Below Basic	9	24	41

■ Below Basic ■ Basic ▨ Intermediate ☐ Proficient

FIGURE 51.ADULT HEALTHCARE LITERACY BY RACE AND ETHNICITY. SOURCE: US DEPT. OF EDUCATION 2003 [270]

Healthcare providers can receive training in how to communicate clearly and effectively, but improving health literacy among patients is critical and currently one of the goals of the Healthy People 2020 initiative and other organizations' efforts. [274]

Language proficiency and health literacy go hand in hand. Patients who do not speak English as their primary language or those who speak Spanish at home are less likely than others to receive preventive care, more likely to struggle with their medications, and require more visits to the office to meet their needs. A patient will not understand instructions if they are provided in a foreign language. Adults who speak only English before starting school have higher health literacy than adults who speak other languages alone or in addition to English.

Average health literacy scores of adults, by race/ethnicity: 2003

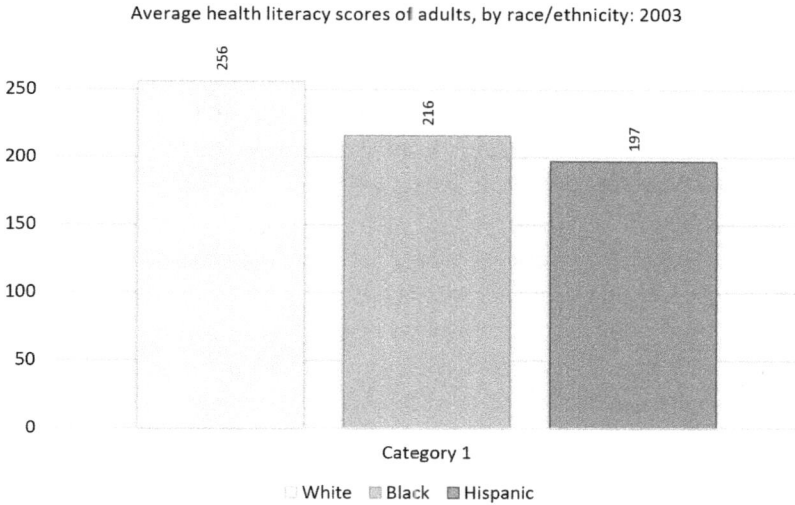

FIGURE 52. AVERAGE HEALTH LITERACY SCORES OF ADULTS, BY RACE/ETHNICITY: 2003

According to the U.S. Census Bureau, **more than 500,000 physicians speak only English at home. In contrast, only 50,000 report speaking Spanish at home**. This demonstrates the scarcity of physicians who are fluent in Spanish and thus able to seamlessly communicate with patients who speak Spanish only.

Patients with limited English proficiency often receive poorer quality care and have worse access to care than fluent patients.

One survey [275] administered in both English and Spanish compared two groups of mostly Hispanic patients. One group reported having poor English skills or using a translator. The second group reported not using a translator and having good English skills. The survey evaluated knowledge on side effects of medications, satisfaction with care, use of preventive tests and feeling that their doctors care for them as patients. Patients with poor English skills were less likely to say that the side effects of their medications were explained to them, which is an issue for compliance with medications that can lead to more frequent hospitalizations. [276-278] They also reported lower patient satisfaction and were less likely to say that the doctors understood how they felt, although the difference was not statistically significant. [275]

These results have been reproduced by other groups. For example, one study of more than 2,000 patients, 50% of whom were Hispanic [279] found not only lower satisfaction with care, more problems with testing, and more difficulties communicating with their providers, but non-English speakers were also less willing to come back to the same emergency room service if they were not satisfied with their care or had problems communicating with their providers.

Other studies have shown that patients treated by language discordant physicians are more likely to omit medication, miss office appointments and make more visits to the emergency room than patients being treated by language concordant physicians. This has implications not only on the prognosis of the patients, but on the cost of health care overall. These findings have been reported in multiple settings such as treatment of asthma patients in the emergency room and delays in the signing of informed consents leading to delayed surgical procedures. [280, 281]

One study assessed the effects of ethnicity and language concordance between patients and physicians on health outcomes, use of health services among Hispanic and non-Hispanic, Spanish-speaking and non-Spanish-speaking patients with hypertension or diabetes. Of the 74 Spanish-speaking Hispanics, 60% were treated by clinicians who spoke Spanish. Having a language-concordant physician was associated with better patient self-reported physical functioning, psychological well-being, health perceptions, and lower pain, and this finding was true even after controlling for patients' age, presence of other medical conditions and prescribed medications, among other potential confounding factors. They also found higher patient satisfaction with care and higher adherence to treatment plans when the physician shared not only the same language, but the same cultural background. [282] As may be expected, these findings are not exclusive to the Hispanic population, but are true for other minority populations as well. [283]

Modern technologies such as tele-health and electronic translation services are helping to address language barriers because they facilitate access to professionals who speak Spanish or other languages and who work "on-demand" to provide interpretation services. Even though extensive data on their effectiveness is not yet available, their help is recommended in circumstances in which language barriers can influence the quality of the health care provided.

Translation and Transcreation

There is increased tension and difficulty in decision-making as well as concerns around legal privacy for providers when family members act as translators. Even though interpretation is often available, particularly in large and urban healthcare centers, this is not always the case in smaller or more rural settings. In addition, words and expressions specific to certain countries or regions can be difficult to understand even for an experienced interpreter. This is why family a member is sometimes preferred as an interpreter, even if the family member is a child who speaks the language fluently (depending on their age and level of health literacy). It's been reported that children tend to have higher levels of health literacy than their parents, and because they are accustomed to serving as interpreters, they tend to have interpreting skills that are more advanced than what would be expected for their age. [284]

One important consideration is that simply translating from English to Spanish is not sufficient. The term "transcreation" is often used in the context of health information materials to refer to a process by which the information is not simply rendered from one language to the other (translation), but the emotional context is taken into account (creation). The goal is to make the receiver of the materials feel the same emotions as the original receiver. Transcreation of medical education materials usually involves the participation of groups of people (focus groups) who are native speakers and who can reach consensus regarding the use of specific words or expressions that convey the desired meaning and trigger the desired reactions or calls to action, such as to undergo a medical procedure, or follow certain treatment instructions. Community participation and input is important when transcreating materials, conducting research and educating healthcare providers. [285]

Again, this is important because some expressions do not have the same meaning in all Spanish-speaking countries and can lead to gross misinterpretation of the materials. One great example of successful transcreation of medical materials include the "Cancer 101" curriculum used to train Master of Public Health students to educate Puerto Rican communities. [286]

Transcreation can also be interpreted as "cultural adaptation" or "cultural targeting" of information towards specific audiences. Some examples of this related to the Hispanic population in particular include a decision aid for Hispanic women. Decision aids are essentially ways to convey information that helps patients make decisions related to serious diseases such as cancer or diabetes, which are associated with high stress and uncertainty levels. These studies have found that involving family members in the decision-making process is more appropriate among Hispanic women, and results in more effective preparation for women making important healthcare-related decisions. [287]

A similar approach has been used among Hispanic male cancer survivors by culturally adapting a tool that measures unmet needs within this patient population. The process of adaptation involved focus groups with patients, providers, psychometric analyses and different types of interviewing techniques aimed at ensuring that the content, the semantics, and the technical aspects of the tool were most appropriate. This is a great example of a process that takes not only language, but culture, literacy and patient needs into account. [288]

Patient-physician racial concordance

Do Hispanics choose to consult physicians of their own race or ethnicity and do non-White physicians provide a disproportionate share of care to underserved populations?

Many factors, including geographic proximity, insurance coverage, and the presence of a physician who speaks their language, influence patients' decisions regarding where to seek care.

A survey that included 542 Hispanics who had regular physicians investigated whether their choice of doctor was influenced by the physician's race and ethnicity or by his or her ability to speak the respondent's language. Black and Hispanic Americans did indeed seek care from physicians of their own race because of personal preference and language, not solely because of geographic accessibility. [289] As many as 42% of Hispanic respondents reported choosing their doctor because of their ability to speak Spanish. The authors state that even though language appears to be a major factor, other factors are clearly at play. One that had been proposed by others is precisely that of cultural sensitivity.

Another important finding of the survey was that even though only 4% of all physicians were Hispanic, they cared for 23% of Hispanic patients. This may be in part due to geographical location, but patient preference is a major factor. [289]

In a recent review publication, the authors analyzed 199 articles related to underrepresented physicians and support for vulnerable patient populations and concluded that even though literature on the topic is lacking and assessments are highly complex; minority patients are more likely to choose a URM (Under Represented Minority) physician and are more satisfied with their care when it is provided by a URM physician. [219, 290]

In three individual studies, Lopez et al showed that Mexican American college students have a clear preference for ethnically similar mental health counselors or psychotherapists. [291] This is independent of the student's gender, knowledge of the objectives of the research, and history of seeking counseling themselves.

One study used the 1990 AMA Physician Masterfile to determine the numbers of physicians practicing in California communities, the 1990 U.S. Census to determine the demographic characteristics of each area, and also surveyed 718 primary care physicians from 51 California communities in 1993 to examine the relation between the physicians' race or ethnic group and the characteristics of the patients they served. Hispanic physicians practiced in areas where the percentage of Hispanic residents was twice as high as areas where other physicians practiced. After controlling for the racial and ethnic makeup of the community, Hispanic physicians cared for significantly more **Hispanic patients and more uninsured patients than did other physicians**. [118]

A study analyzing data from the National Medical Expenditure Survey, which provides national estimates of healthcare utilization and expenditures, concluded that non-White physicians are more likely to care for minority, medically indigent, and sicker patients. **Minority patients were more than four times more likely to receive care from non-White physicians when compared with non-Hispanic White patients**. These patients are more likely to report worse health, have chronic conditions, psychological disorders and be hospitalized, which the authors suggest may penalize non-White physicians. [292]

Using data for 48,388 physicians, Walker et al found that African American, Latino, and Pacific Islanders were more likely to work in MUAs and HPSAs than were White physicians. [293]

Another survey asked the question of whether patient-physician racial concordance affects patient satisfaction with and use of health care. The majority of Hispanic respondents were Mexican or Puerto Rican. Hispanic patients did not rate Hispanic physicians differently from non-Hispanic physicians in terms of treating them with respect or explaining medical issues to them. However, **they were more likely to be very satisfied with their health care overall when they had a Hispanic doctor**. [294]

One more study reported data from a cross-sectional analysis of 7,070 adults in the 2010 Medical Expenditure Panel Survey in which the authors estimated the likelihood of having a non-White physician for patients who were racial and ethnic minorities, low income, Medicaid enrollees, uninsured, and non-English home language speakers. Non-White physicians were more likely to practice primary care and to care for minority patients, including those from communities with lower socioeconomic status. The investigators adjusted for confounding factors such as geographical location, type of office, physician sex and others. **They found that non-White physicians cared for 53.5% of minority and 70.4% of non–English-speaking patients, and that patients from underserved groups were significantly more likely to see non-White physicians than White physicians**. [295]

According to the National Survey of Early Care and Education, [296] high-Hispanic-serving centers are more likely to help children and families access comprehensive services such as developmental assessments, social services, health screenings and access to specialists. Centers serving high percentages of young Hispanic children compare favorably to other centers on key predictors of quality.

Physician bias and racial variations in the use of treatments and procedures

Explicit bias refers to negative or positive attitudes that include "thoughts and feelings that people deliberately think about and can consciously report about." In contrast, implicit racial biases refer to the subconscious, often automatic attitudes towards members of different racial/ethnic groups, of which the individual is often unaware and would not explicitly express.

It has been proposed that due to anxiety surrounding their own ability to engage with individuals of a different race or who speak another language, White physicians may subconsciously display avoidant behaviors when interacting with non-White patients, leading to deficiencies in physician-patient communication.

According to the Institute of Medicine, even when insured at the same level, minority populations receive lower quality care and fewer healthcare services.

Hispanic patients seen in emergency care settings have been shown to be less likely to receive analgesia and this is true even after controlling for language spoken. [297-299]

A five-year retrospective analysis was conducted in Florida to quantify the number of major complications among adult patients who were admitted to hospitals with diagnoses such as sepsis, surgical site infection, pulmonary embolism, acute renal failure, myocardial infarction, cerebrovascular accident, and pneumonia. More than half a million cases were analyzed, which included more than 5,000 surgeons and more than 200 hospitals. [300] 14.2% of the patients included in the study were Hispanic. One-fifth of the surgeons were considered "low-minority treating" (LM), while 9.4% were "high-minority treating" (HM). The majority of Hispanic patients (70.6%) did not receive their care from HM surgeons. **The analysis showed that non-White patients had overall higher odds of sustaining a major complication, but Black and Hispanic patients had lower risk-adjusted odds of complications when treated by HM surgeons, even after controlling for hospital facility characteristics.** Even though the group of Black and Hispanic patients treated by

LM surgeons was small, adjusted analysis showed higher odds of complications, although these results were not significant The results suggest that HM surgeons may be better able to provide high quality, safe care to non-White patients.

The authors hypothesized that HM surgeons are more comfortable engaging with non-White patients and better able to communicate effectively, build trust and counsel the patients, which leads to an overall improved quality of care. They also proposed that perhaps their frequent interaction with non-White patients helps them be more attuned to the prejudices related to healthcare inequities, which makes them more aware of their own implicit racial biases, which results in better care. In fact, it's been reported that denying the unconscious bias is a key characteristic of "aversive" racism, a subconscious attitude held by people who outwardly express egalitarian values and justify their behaviors by factors other than race, such as genetic predisposition among Hispanics and Blacks.

Participation in research and access to novel and investigational treatments

Minority populations participate in clinical research as human subjects less frequently than nonminority populations in spite of the fact that some minorities experience the same or higher rates of some of the diseases under investigation than Whites.

There are numerous tools used in medicine to assess a patient's response to an intervention. These tools are known as "outcome measures." Some examples include: the number of patients responding to an experimental treatment, the impact of a disease on a patient's quality of life, the percentage of patients who survived after a transplant, etc.

Research involving ethnic minority populations requires cultural and linguistically appropriate methodologies. Many outcome measures are translated into Spanish without taking into account cultural differences, regional language nuances, literacy, age of the target patient population and other factors. Taking these factors into account results in improved comprehension and acceptability of the tools, potentially resulting in more accurate data collection.

Participation in research would also help us decipher the mysterious "Latino paradox" by which first-generation Hispanics have a better health status than Whites and second and third-generation Hispanics living in the U.S.

Can cultural and linguistic competence be taught and measured?

Since 2000, the Liaison Committee on Medical Education (LCME) introduced a standard for cultural competence education in medical schools: "The faculty and students must demonstrate an understanding of the manner in which people of diverse cultures and belief systems perceive health and illness and respond to various symptoms, diseases, and treatments. Medical students should learn to recognize and appropriately address gender and cultural biases in healthcare delivery, while considering first the health of the patient."

Cultural competence is now taught in many medical schools, hospitals, clinics and other healthcare environments. Different modalities of training are being implemented, including some that are led by the students themselves, with good results. [301]

However, few studies demonstrate the benefit of cultural competence training on patient health outcomes, [302-304] perhaps because education on this topic has only recently been implemented and it is still not clear what type of training is most effective, or how to evaluate its effectiveness both at the individual and institutional level, as well as among leaders. [305, 306]

Even though some of the existing data does suggest that biases may be "malleable" and can be "unlearned" [307], and that cultural competence training does lead to increased knowledge and confidence among healthcare practitioners and improved patient satisfaction with the clinical encounter [308, 309], short workshop-type education, as well as other forms of small-scale trainings appear to be effective immediately after the intervention, but not in the long-term.

Most importantly, patient outcomes appear not to be significantly affected significantly by cultural competence training. [306, 309, 310] Many have labeled this type of training as "Latino 101" crash courses that do teach physicians to be more aware of cultural and linguistic differences and barriers, but does not prepare them for the tremendous diversity that they deal with every day and could even be considered impractical and even divisive. [309, 310]

Interventions to increase health literacy among immigrants have also shown mixed results. In a systematic review, Fernandez-Gutierrez et al. [311] showed that most published studies either report on inadequate sample sizes (too few patients) or use instruments that have not been validated to measure health literacy outcomes appropriately. Out of the few scientifically sound studies identified, most showed an increase in functional health literacy, which means increased knowledge and understanding of the information, but less of an impact on actual behaviors. More research is needed on this topic.

Linguistic competence is even more difficult to implement broadly. As mentioned before, the Centers for Medicare & Medicaid Services (CMS) recommends providing appropriate oral and written language services through bilingual/bicultural staff, trained medical interpreters, and qualified translators. **There is recognition of the fact that a provider who does not speak the language will not be able to provide both oral and written language services to limited English proficiency patients**.

One alternative is to identify linguistically competent physicians proactively to make sure that they are available when needed. In a study conducted in California [312] the researchers validated a simple questionnaire that identifies language-competent physicians. Interestingly, a single, self-reported proficiency question provided a fast, low cost, reasonably accurate way for a healthcare institution to assess Spanish Medical proficiency.

One could argue that self-reported proficiency is subjective, and indeed the validation results do show relatively low correlations between medical proficiency and patient reports. In addition, those language-competent physicians should get certified to avoid negative outcomes. The Agency for Healthcare Research and Quality (AHRQ) has developed guidelines regarding the participation of language-competent staff members. [313] These tools and clear protocols should at the very least, allow for Institutions applying this simple questionnaire to identify physicians who are more apt than the rest to treat Spanish-speaking patients, reducing the risks and costs associated with patient interactions with physicians who are not linguistically competent. [314]
However, based on the demographic data presented in this book, it is clear that a sufficient number of Spanish-speaking physicians is not available to fulfill this need.

As many other authors have stated, the purpose of these comments is not to disparage cultural competence education, which is desperately needed. Instead, I am trying to highlight the fact that it is difficult to teach and that many of the current models of cultural and linguistic competence education do not appear to change long-term behaviors or decisions that affect patient outcomes.

Teaching cultural and linguistic competence is difficult, and most of the available data fails to demonstrate significant benefits in patient outcomes. This may be because cultural competence training tends to be superficial and short.

Choosing a healthcare provider and communicating information about one's health to him or her is a very delicate and personal matter. As others have said, data to explain why racial-concordance in the patient-physician encounter matter so much is lacking, perhaps simply because it is impossible to measure the emotional aspects of that encounter. If we were able to measure it and understand it, we would teach the entire workforce how to achieve those outcomes.

There are two ways to address this gap. First, cultural competence education must be re-evaluated and new, more robust and more consistent methods of training must be put in place. Second, efforts to increase the diversity in the health professions will allow for a sufficient number of physicians matching the diversity of the general population who are available to treat patients of their own culture and language appropriately.

In the next section, I summarize several examples of culturally and linguistically appropriate programs that address the most common causes of death as well as the most impactful conditions from the quality of life point of view.

Application of culturally and linguistically competent care among Hispanic patients

The Starr Country Border Health Initiative was a culturally competent diabetes self-management intervention that enrolled 256 Mexican Americans ages 35-70 with a diagnosis of Type 2 diabetes and randomized half of them to the intervention and the other half to a control arm. 97.7% of Starr County, TX inhabitants were Mexican American. Importantly, the study also enrolled one close family member as a support person. Bilingual researchers conducted phone and in-person interviews making an effort to make participants feel comfortable, reading questions aloud in Spanish and English, and avoiding judgment of participant's health practices such as alternative medicine. The intervention also included instruction sessions for individuals and their support persons. 90% of participants chose Spanish as their preferred language and 78% spoke Spanish at home. Among the outcome measures were diabetes knowledge, fasting blood glucose (FBG) and HbA1c, which is a test that allows physicians to get an overall picture of what our average blood sugar levels have been over a period of weeks/months. The higher the HbA1c, the greater the risk of developing diabetes-related complications. Among the key results of the intervention were an improvement in diabetes knowledge of 14.4% from baseline in the intervention group, as compared to a 4.8% improvement in the control group and statistically significant differences between the two groups on FBG and HbA1c levels. [315, 316]

Cuidando el Corazon was a culturally adapted weight-reduction and exercise program for Mexican Americans, also in Texas. The program enrolled women, 18-45 years of age, with at least one child and who were >20% above the ideal weight. Most of them had a family income of about $20,000 and an average education attainment of tenth grade. Participants were divided into three groups that were exposed to different intervention modalities. One group received a manual with behavioral and nutritional advice, a second group received the same manual in addition to year-long class attendance, and a third group received a family intervention to address family eating and exercise habits. The project had a high attrition rate, and even though the majority of the participants did not achieve significant changes in their weight, the greatest weight loss occurred in the family group. This highlights the importance of family engagement in interventions targeting low-income minority participants [317]

Hispanics living in California, also suffer from a high prevalence of Type 2 diabetes. Lumetra, the Medicare quality improvement organization for California, developed the **Viva Su Vida** (Live Your Life) program. A three-year project to improve diabetes care for Medicare beneficiaries of Hispanic origin, to help decrease the disparity in HbA1c testing rates between White and Latino beneficiaries in 4 counties. The materials created included a booklet directed to patients and their families with easy-to-understand graphics, a card with sample questions to facilitate patient-physician interactions and to record test results, a colorful sheet listing all supplies and services covered by Medicare, and a resource guide for providers including a section on cultural competence. Even though the disparity had started to narrow during the years prior to the intervention, the Viva Su Vida program is thought to have helped to narrow the disparity further from a 7.1% difference between White and Hispanic testing rates, to 3.0% at the end of the intervention. [318]

The **Secretos de la Buena Vida** project evaluated Hispanic women after different types of intervention ranging from face-to-face visits by health advisors to mailed information pieces on nutrition. Groups receiving the face-to-face intervention showed significantly lower levels of total fat and carbohydrate intake. Married women were four times more likely to adopt dietary fat changes than single women. Although the changes were not long-lasting, the study demonstrated the importance of the interpersonal interaction in the behavioral change. [319, 320] Hispanic women appear to need a higher number of visits or other modes of interpersonal interaction (e.g. phone calls) to adopt a behavioral change. [321]

A group of researchers from the University of California conducted cultural and linguistic adaptation of healthy diet text messages. The group translated **HealthyYouTXT**, which is a program designed to send users five texts a day for several weeks to promote healthy dietary practices. The program was developed by the National Cancer Institute and is available free of charge to continental U.S. residents. Content for this type of tool tends to be developed through research conducted mainly among non-Hispanic participants and thus, the theoretical framework is based on beliefs and values that may not be necessarily relevant to the Hispanic population. Some examples listed by the authors include: familialism (i.e. prioritizing family values over your own), destiny (beliefs that outcomes are destined to occur), among others. The researchers went on to incorporate some of these concepts into the statements in the text messages by introducing information about the benefits of healthy eating for the whole family, or by suggesting family meals to address familialism. Importantly, the researchers revised the text libraries to enhance their cultural appropriateness and to address generational and belief systems divergences based on participants' feedback. For instance, younger Hispanics preferred the use of *tu* instead of used. They also used "Pan-American words" to make the language accessible to most Spanish speakers e.g. *platano* instead of *guineo* or *banano*. An interesting and very informative example was the use of the expression *comida chatarra* to refer to junk food. Most participants found the Spanish expression inappropriate and even recommended the use of the term in English instead. Finally, the use of Spanish grammatical symbols appeared to increase the credibility of the messages. Overall, this interesting study demonstrates the importance of thoughtful linguistic and cultural adaptation of materials developed with the help of non-Hispanic participants. [322]

Some other programs worth reviewing, especially if they're in your area are the following:

- Latino Health for All Coalition programs, including Wyandotte Deserves, which provides access to healthy food and physical activity to Latinos in Wyandotte County in Kansas:, the Diabetes prevention program, which provides education and screening services and the Cultural Competence Project, which provides training sessions and workshops directed to healthcare organizations.
- The Latino Health Outreach Project from the Institute for Family Health in New York. Multiple publications of interest are available on their website. I particularly recommend the following article on factors needed to guide future efforts to eliminate racial/ethnic disparities in diabetes control. [249]
- The Montgomery County Latino Health initiative, a culturally and linguistically competent health wellness system for Latinos, serving a population with low levels of health insurance and low English proficiency.
- Proyecto Salud, which seeks to provide high quality, culturally competent, and affordable primary healthcare services to its patients in Maryland.

Celebremos la Salud (Celebrating Health), was a program to increase awareness and improve health habits related to colorectal, breast and cervical cancer, as well as nutrition and smoking among rural communities comprised primarily of Hispanics. Even though the study found more awareness of and participation in intervention activities in the intervention group than the control group, there were no significant differences in use of screening tests for cervical (Pap test), breast (mammogram) or colorectal cancer (fecal occult blood test [FOBT] or colonoscopy) between the two groups. [323]

These results demonstrate a sad truth that contradicts the theoretical expectation. **Increased knowledge does not always result in increased intention**. In other words, even when an intervention results in increased awareness about risk factors and management of a specific disease, low-income participants who lack health insurance are unable to take action. In fact, these were the conclusions from a post-hoc study that was conducted to determine reasons for lack of effectiveness of the **Celebremos la Salud** intervention. In the study report, the authors found that having participated in live presentations at organizations was the only activity that positively correlated with breast cancer testing in the last two years, but that the lack of success of the intervention was likely related to the fact that many of the participants were Hispanic women with low educational attainment and no health insurance. [324]

Although marginally significant, other studies support the need for face-to-face, group-based interventions in order to obtain changes in a participant's intention to obtain a mammogram and other cancer screening tests after the intervention. One approach that appears to be particularly useful is the engagement of health promotores (bilingual and bicultural community health workers) which increases the understanding of the information and ... social interaction. [325-328]
One example of a successful promotoras-based intervention, **Las Mujeres Saludables** (Healthy Women) was a 12-week program working with promotoras that recruited 366 Hispanic women from community-based organizations and educated them in breast, cervical and colorectal cancer prevention and screening while emphasizing social support among class members. Some of the positive

outcomes of this intervention included an increase in physical activity from 65.15 to 122.40 minutes/week and more than 30% of participants undergoing Pap tests and mammograms. [329]

The Tepeyac Project was a church-based health promotion project to increase breast cancer screening rates among Hispanic women in Colorado. The program included either printed education packages or promotoras delivering breast-health education messages personally. As with other similar programs described here, the promotoras method resulted in slightly, but not statistically significantly better outcomes than the printed packages. However, the overall conclusion was that regardless of the insurance status, education alone may not be the answer for this population. [330, 331]

Data from more than 500 Latinas that had participated in the programs Women and Cancer and Nutrition and Cancer, which were part of the *Por la Vida* project in San Diego, CA, showed significant increases in the frequency of Pap testing among women participating in the Women and Cancer program, compared to no changes among those participating in the Nutrition and Cancer program, which did not include Pap test-specific information. The intervention included education provided by community health workers. [332, 333]

Another multifaceted program named **A Su Salud** (To Your health), led by University Health System in Texas and funded by the Cancer Prevention & Research Institute of Texas (CPRIT) [334], is aimed at increasing awareness around nutrition, cancer and injury prevention, among other topics. It started as a smoking cessation program in 1984, and it primarily seeks to improve health-related behaviors in populations with limited access to medical information and healthcare services. Based on social cognitive theory, one central approach has been the use of health advisors to recruit participants to join them in listening or watching television or radio programs on specific topics and then having a discussion with the participants to improve understanding and reinforce key messages. Another approach is the use of social media, newsletters and public service announcements to reach out to more than one million Texan residents. The part of the program focusing on colorectal cancer screening enrolled Hispanic men who had never received a colonoscopy and resulted in more than 300 men screened. Almost half of them had polyps that could have led to colorectal cancer, demonstrating the tremendous value of this type of program.

The National Cancer Institute conducted a program to increase the reach of culturally competent smoking cessation counseling among Spanish-speaking smokers. The program was named **Adios al Fumar** (Goodbye to Smoking). The program used targeted promotion, and in spite of the fact that most participants were of low socioeconomic status—a population that is considered hard to reach—they were able to increase the number of calls to the Cancer Information Service (CIS) from 0.39 to 17.8%. [335] A survey conducted in the early 2000's through the CIS found that Hispanics had the highest level of awareness of the CIS language among all racial and ethnic groups included. [336]

Another family-based intervention to prevent tobacco and alcohol use among migrant Hispanic youth funded by the National Cancer Institute was **Sembrando Salud** (Sowing Health). It was an eight-session, culturally sensitive program presented by bilingual/bicultural college students. Parents attended three of the eight sessions helping their child complete homework assignments. The content of the treatment intervention included information about tobacco and alcohol effects, training on refusal skills, and parent-child communication skills to support healthy decisions. Unfortunately the intervention was not shown to be effective, which the authors hypothesized may be related to the low rates of smoking and drinking even prior to the intervention. [337]

Other studies have shown that the percentage of Hispanic women counseled about Pap tests in 2015 was lower (49.4%, age-adjusted, 21–65 years) compared to White women (54.3%). In other words, the rate of Pap test counseling in the White, non-Hispanic population is 11% higher than the rate for the Hispanic or Latino population.

One example of a culturally-sensitive intervention was the use of educational videos played in waiting rooms, which resulted in an increase in the proportion of women obtaining Pap smears after the intervention. [338, 339]

A similar approach was used when including breast cancer educational content in a popular telenovela (soap opera) titled **Ladrón de Corazones**. This intervention resulted in an increase in the number of calls to the information line 1-800-4-cancer when the number was featured during the broadcast. In addition, a survey conducted after the intervention showed increased knowledge on the topic nationwide. [340]

Nueva Vida is an ongoing program that was founded in 1996 by Latina breast cancer survivors as a partnership between the community and academia to provide culturally sensitive support to cancer patients in the Washington D.C. area. The program has published data form several studies that can be found on their website. One example is a study using formal outcome measures of quality of life, self-effectiveness (i.e. The Cancer Behavior Inventory), and psychological distress, during the course of one year while the enrollees received individual counseling, participated in support groups and engaged in peer support. [341]

Numerous other articles have been published on the topic of breast cancer interventions among Hispanic women and I encourage interested readers to review the following references, and to visit the website for the Conference on The Science of Cancer Health Disparities in Racial/Ethnic Minorities and the Medically Underserved from the American Association of Cancer Research. [327, 342]

Among male Hispanics, the most common type of cancer is prostate cancer but lung cancer results in the most deaths. Thus, interventions focusing on early prostate cancer diagnosis and smoking cessation are key.

In terms of the percentage of men ever counseled about advantages and disadvantages of the PSA test for prostate cancer detection (age-adjusted, 40+ years), White non-Hispanic or Latino rates were 32.9% higher than the rate for the Hispanic or Latino population. The rate of prostate cancer deaths (age-adjusted, per 100,000 population) for Hispanics was 15.4 in 2017, versus 17.8 for Whites and 36.8 for African Americans.

Reproductive and sexual health

Infosida (AIDSinfo) is a website from the National Institutes of Health (NIH) with extensive information on terminology related to HIV, treatments available, testing, clinical trials and clinical guidelines both in English and Spanish.

The **Center for Latino Adolescent and Family Health** (CLAFH), with programs to support communication between parents and teens, promotes healthy behaviors including tobacco and drug use avoidance, and even family economic wellbeing education.

Numerous programs have been put into place to help decrease the number of teen pregnancies. Even though not all of them have specifically targeted Hispanic adolescents—who have the highest rates of pregnancy of all races and ethnicities—many have been translated using culturally appropriate methodologies.

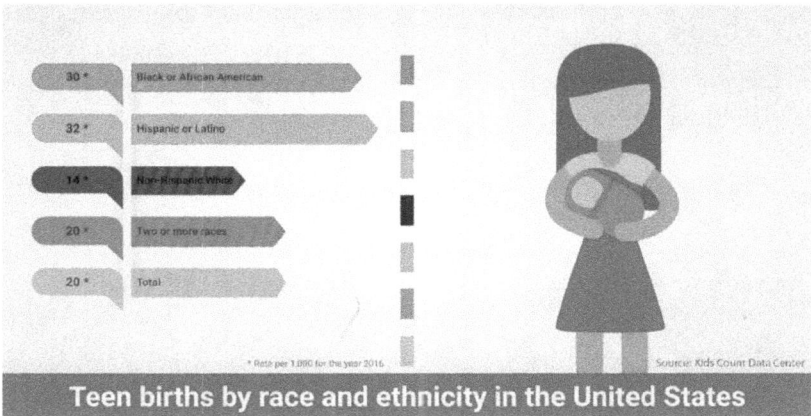

FIGURE 53. TEEN BIRTHS BY RACE AND ETHNICITY IN THE U.S.

All4you is a 26-hour long program to prevent HIV, other STD and pregnancy among students in grades 9–12 in alternative education settings.

¡Cuidate! Is a 6-module culturally based curriculum designed to reduce HIV sexual risk specifically among Latino youth.

A list of many available programs focusing on teen pregnancy prevention has been put together by the Office of Adolescent health and can be found in this website: https://www.hhs.gov/ash/oah/sites/default/files/ebp-chart1.pdf

Key takeaways from chapter 6

1

Talking about something as serious and intimate as your own health is easier when the healthcare provider is able to communicate and understand you, as well as relate to you culturally.

2

Cultural competence acknowledges variations in customs, traditions, values, beliefs, and communication styles and takes them into account when assessing and treating individuals.

3

A culturally competent professional provides information and services in the language, as well as in the educational and cultural context most appropriate for the individuals he or she serves.

4

Cultural and linguistic competence are particularly relevant when communicating health-related information to a population with low health literacy. Health literacy allows patients to understand their conditions and the treatments that will improve their overall well-being. Hispanic adults have the lowest average health literacy score compared to adults in other racial and ethnic groups.

5

Translating medical information from English to Spanish is not sufficient. The term "transcreation" refers to a process by which the information is not simply rendered from one language to the other (translation), but the emotional context is taken into account (creation). Transcreation can also be interpreted as "cultural adaptation" of the materials.

6

A patient's satisfaction with the clinical encounter increases when the physician has similar racial/ethnic and linguistic backgrounds. A physician's race and language influences the choice of physician that Hispanic patients make.

7

Almost half of Hispanic patients choose their physician not only based on insurance coverage and geographical proximity, but also based on the physician's ability to speak their language.

8

Non-White physicians provide a disproportionate share of care to underserved populations but there is a shortage of Hispanic physicians in areas with high concentration of Hispanics.

9

Cultural competence training programs are in place in medical schools and in many institutions, but there is limited evidence that proves that short "crash courses" in cultural competence make a difference in patient outcomes. Even though this does not mean that these programs should not be conducted, their content and duration need to be carefully evaluated.

10

Increased knowledge does not always result in increased intention. Even when an intervention results in increased awareness about risk factors and management of a specific disease, low-income participants who lack health insurance, have low health literacy or have no access to a culturally and linguistically competent physician are unable to take action.

11

Equal representation of Hispanic physicians in the health care workforce is the best solution to ensure that a sufficient number of culturally and linguistically competent physicians are available to address the needs of the Hispanic population.

Online resources for chapter 6

IF YOU ARE INTERESTED IN:	GO TO:
Cultural and linguistic competence training for physicians	U.S. Department of Health & Human Services https://www.hhs.gov/ash/oah/resources-and-training/tpp-and-paf-resources/cultural-competence/index.html https://thinkculturalhealth.hhs.gov/education/behavioral-health Michigan Technological University's Center for Diversity and Inclusion (CDI) https://www.mtu.edu/diversity-center/programs/competency/ University of Wisconsin- Population Health Institute with funding from the Robert Johnson Foundation https://www.countyhealthrankings.org/take-action-to-improve-health/what-works-for-health/strategies/cultural-competence-training-for-health-care-professionals
AAMC- Tool for Assessing Cultural Competence Training (TACCT)	https://www.aamc.org/what-we-do/mission-areas/diversity-inclusion/tool-for-assessing-cultural-competence-training

| Podcast on disparities in health care | Dismantling Disparities in Health Care https://anchor.fm/disparitiessolutions |

STORIES OF HISPANIC PHYSICIANS AND SCIENTISTS IN THE U.S.

ANA MARIA DOES NOT HAVE MENTORS OR ROLE MODELS

"Doctor, can I ask you another question?"

"Yes of course, Ana Maria, what is it?"

"Have you ever met a Hispanic doctor?"

"Of course I have! As a matter of fact, a close friend of mine in medical school was from Peru, his name is Juan. I haven't seen him in a long time. He went to practice in a remote area on the Mexican-American border after residency and I never saw him again."

"Were his parents rich?"

"That's an odd question! Do you think the only way to go to med school is if you're wealthy? My parents were very poor. I kept trying until I found a school that gave me a grant instead of a loan and that's how I was able to go to medical school. I also worked nights for years to save money for school and so did my mom. Remember what Walt Disney used to say, 'If you can dream it, you can do it!'"

A renewed feeling of hope filled Ana Maria's heart, as she walked next to her sister and mother out of the hospital.

Ana Maria makes an important observation during her conversation with her sister's doctor. She has never met a Hispanic physician.

According to the Pew Research Center, [343] when asked, "In your opinion, who is the most important Hispanic/Latino leader in the country today?," most Hispanics (62%) say that they don't know and 9% say "no one." Yet most of them say that it is very important or extremely important for the community to have one.

In chapter 4 I talked about the critical importance of mentorship in educational outcomes. In this section, I wanted to share stories of Hispanic physicians in the U.S. and I'm grateful to those who agreed to contribute. I sincerely hope that they inspire you in the same manner as they inspired me.

ARTURO CASADEVALL

Arturo Casadevall, M.D., Ph.D. is a Bloomberg Distinguished Professor of Molecular Microbiology & Immunology and Infectious Diseases at the Johns Hopkins Bloomberg School of Public Health and Johns Hopkins School of Medicine and Alfred and Jill Sommer Professor and Chair of the W. Harry Feinstone Department of Molecular Microbiology and Immunology at the Johns Hopkins Bloomberg School of Public Health.

Dr. Casadevall has served as President of the Medical Mycology Society of America, Chair of American Society for Microbiology Division, Chair of the American Society for Microbiology Career Development Committee, and Co-Chair of the National Institute of Allergy and Infectious Diseases Board of Scientific Counselors, and currently serves on the Scientific Council of the Pasteur Institute.

In 2014, he became an elected member of the National Academy of Medicine and in 2017, he was elected to the American Academy of Arts and Sciences. Dr. Casadevall was the first Hispanic Department Chair at the Albert Einstein College of Medicine.

What can you tell us about your personal journey?
I'm a Cuban exile. I came to the U.S. when I was 11 years-old. We were poor. There were eight of us living at an apartment in Elmhurst, Queens. However, my family always held the deep belief that education was a ticket to success. This may be why I decided to focus on education, to get away from that situation.

Where did you go to school and how did you overcome the monetary and language limitations?
I discovered science in high school. I couldn't believe that people got paid to do research so I decided that I wanted to go for a career in science.

With regards to language, I didn't speak English well at all, and maybe for that reason, I did best in math and chemistry. I applied myself to get the best grades that I could get. The idea that education was my ticket to get out of my circumstances served as my motivation.

My family didn't have money for me to go to college. I could not even consider Stony Brook, part of the State University of New York, which would have been a natural option due to its location. However, City University of New York was an option. The first year was free and then you payed tuition. I worked four nights a week thorough college to be able to cover the cost. I was a blood-drawer at the Veterans Administration. I used to leave Queens at 4:00 am to be able to get to work by 6:00 am. I heard that the supervisor was Cuban-Asian, so I figured that she would be willing to give me a chance. I had never drawn blood, but she taught me. I received my B.A. in Chemistry from CUNY.

Was your family supportive of your career choice?
My father didn't pay much attention to what I was doing. He had been a lawyer in Cuba. When I told him that I had been accepted to the Chemistry program at Columbia University, he did not truly understand the implications. A common issue with Hispanic parents is the lack of understanding of the career options for their kids. There is also a tendency to elevate patient care over research. As a matter of fact, when my father realized that I was doing well, he told me that I should go to Medical School.

I studied all summer to make it into premed. One day, I found out that there was a combined MD/PhD program at New York University, which I thought was the best of both worlds. However, I was warned that no one from CUNY would be able to get in. I was accepted, but I got in at the last minute. Even though it was not my original intention to pursue a career in medicine, once I started, I loved it. I realized that it was a good thing to do. I did my residency at Bellevue Hospital in New York City.

Did you have a mentor? Can you tell us how he or she helped you get to where you are?
At Queens College Department of Medicine, my English was bad so I really needed help with my essay. I made an appointment to see a professor there. He asked to see the essay and helped tremendously. I found out he was a concentration camp survivor. I wouldn't say that he was my mentor but I am grateful for what he did for

me. He died recently. I did have the opportunity to visit him to thank him before he passed. After that, there were PhD advisors, for instance, who mentor you when you choose a career in science.

Why do you think that so few Hispanics pursue careers in science and medicine?
I actually never had a Hispanic classmates. There were a few at NYU Medical School. Only 25 women out of 170 students and maybe 9 or 10 Hispanics overall.
From the reaction of my father when I told him that this was my career choice, I can say that there seems to be little awareness about careers in research within the Hispanic community. And, as I mentioned before, it seems as if the cultural tradition is patient care, not research.

Why is it important to help increase Latino representation in science and medicine?
Each culture brings different things to the table. Even if the contribution is only 1% different, it brings entirely new insights. Humanity needs that diversity. For instance, drugs don't work the same for all races and ethnicities, and pharmaceutical companies need to conduct clinical trials in specific regions of the world to explore idiosyncratic reactions.

Similarly, each culture brings different ways of doing things. When it comes to creative experiments, Latin American scientists are, in my opinion, particularly creative. I see this when I travel to Latin America to meet with scientists. It's the lack of resources that prevents science in Latin American countries from thriving.

I take a lot of courses from The Teaching Company. One course that I took explored the question of whether South Americans should be considered part of Western culture or whether they are an entirely different culture. We are clearly a younger culture. Remarkably diverse and creative.

Having experienced patient care with Hispanics so closely, how important do you think cultural and linguistic competence is for Hispanics?
I think that language is the main barrier. More than cultural competency and understanding. Language provides a clear, common bond. There are many language nuances that people are not aware of. I have myself have experienced it when I travel to other Spanish-speaking countries where simple, everyday words can have a completely different meaning I also experienced it at Bellevue Hospital where most of the patient population was Hispanic.

What advice do you have for others who want to follow your path?
Well, the world is very different now, compared to when I went to school. Young Hispanic students are better than I ever was. They also have access to a wealth of information and services nowadays. The issue, I think, is that they do not know what opportunities are available to them. It may not be a question of equality. Beyond equality, there's lack of opportunity. It's not a level playing field.

Science is not even on their radar or within their parents' scope of thinking. My father for instance, was disappointed when I told him that I was interested in a career in science. He also had a hard time understanding the opportunity. I remember one of our conversations in our kitchen:

My father: "Do you mean to tell me that you have been admitted to a program in which they will pay **you**?"

Me: "Yes, dad! There is a program where they pay physicians to become scientists."

Two other barriers are time and location. For many Hispanics who need a salary to support their families, the mere idea of a four-year college degree, followed by four years of medical school, four more years of residency and possibly fellowships and other training, is neither practical nor affordable. In terms of location, there are issues that are specific to certain environments. Access to education is an important consideration. I moved to John Hopkins five years ago, and I see differences between where I went to school and this institution.

If you had unlimited resources, what action would you prioritize to help young Hispanics living in the U.S. who are interested in pursuing careers in medicine?
When I was at the Albert Einstein College of Medicine, the school had a very diverse population with large numbers of underrepresented minorities—probably due to its location in the Bronx, New York. The problem was the unacceptably large rates of attrition. Students didn't do very well in courses. The grades that they were being admitted with, didn't match their preparation. I think that everybody should take an exam aimed at identifying their weaknesses. Deficits can be corrected. I would have liked for the school to send them to specific classes to compensate for those deficits. If I received an unrestricted grant, I would help them by creating programs to strengthen their weakest areas.

What book would you recommend to young Hispanic students interested in a career in medicine?

Anna Karenina by Leo Tolstoy. I like it because it is a very rich, detailed book that has a lot to say about the human experience. Even the first sentence in the book: "All happy families are alike; each unhappy family is unhappy in its own way."

Anna Karenina tells you so much about life experiences. I read it in my first year of medical school during those early morning train rides to get to my job as a blood-drawer. I used to think that all graduate students are happy or unhappy in their own way.

What advice do you have for others who want to follow your path?

Do as much as possible to broaden your knowledge of humanity. Science and medicine will always try to specialize you so you must try to be different.

CONSUELO (CONNIE) CASILLAS

Consuelo Casillas, M.D. is Partner at Southern California Permanente Medical Group, Family Physician at Kaiser Permanente Los Angeles Medical Center and Clinical Instructor at Kaiser Permanente Bernard J. Tyson School of Medicine and David Geffen UCLA School of Medicine

Dr. Casillas serves as Executive Board Member for the Alliance in Mentorship, 501c3 for MiMentor and for Latinx Physicians of California

Dr. Casillas was elected Family Physician of the Year at Kaiser Permanente, Los Angeles Medical Center in 2017 and Top Women Leaders in Health Care by the Los Angeles Business Journal in 2020. She received the MiMentor Alma Award for outstanding leadership and inspiration for the next generation of healthcare leaders in 2019.

As a Latina family physician, my ability to reflect cultural values such as "confianza," "respeto," and "familismo" greatly facilitates the doctor-patient relationship. The human experience shared through these relationships is an unparalleled privilege I cherish as a physician. The daily clinical challenges are gratifying, but most importantly, medicine has enriched my life with boundless humility for the human experience. As Latinx populations quickly become a majority-minority across the United States, physician leaders who intimately understand the Latinx experience and can advocate for the needs of our communities are direly needed.

One barrier I've had to overcome in my career is impostorism. Impostorism is the persistent internalized fear of being exposed as a "fraud, or of doubting one's accomplishments. In my particular case, impostorism manifested itself whenever I minimized my accomplishments. This tendency may be rooted in the intersectionality of my gender, culture or other personal traits. In high school, I favored relating to those individuals who were more "street," than "booksmart," and whose academic paths ended at or before high school. Lack of awareness of how to reconcile responsibilities as a mother, partner and physician leader further led to marginalization of my own professional leadership aspirations. I am certain that effective mentorship earlier in my life would have validated my strengths and empowered me to envision new career path possibilities.

During my career, I've seen health care disparities for my patients because of language and/or cultural barriers. To increase the number of physicians who can overcome these barriers, I've worked the past 5 years to mentor young people from medically underserved communities to become doctors, nurses and physician's assistants. With increasing diversity in the U.S., and the simultaneous decrease in the percentage of Latinx healthcare workforce, the urgency of this mentorship is deeply felt by many of my Latinx physician colleagues. With each, *Que Dios me la cuide*, and other words of gratitude from my patients, it strengthens my resolve to focus on mentoring underrepresented in medicine students.

Currently I'm an executive board member and Chief Information Officer for Alliance in Mentorship, the founding entity of MiMentor. MiMentor is a free multi-platform social media network which develops and supports innovative and inclusive mentoring opportunities to inspire the next generation of diverse healthcare leaders for underserved communities (MiMentor.org). I am also an executive board member for Latinx Physicians of California which is also working on programming to build a more equitable healthcare workforce to serve our Latinx communities. I want to inspire younger pre-health professionals through this and other ways that a career in medicine can be extremely fulfilling. And when this new generation becomes our next generation of physicians, nurses and physician assistants, they will also become the diverse leaders our health care system so desperately needs.

JUAN CARLOS CAICEDO

Juan Carlos Caicedo, M.D., is an Associate Professor of Surgery (Organ Transplantation) Director, Hispanic Transplant Program

Surgical Director, Liver Transplant Program and Hepatobiliary Surgery

Director, Living Donor Liver Transplant Program

Transplant Surgeon, Northwestern Memorial Hospital

Pediatric Transplant Surgeon, Lurie Children's Hospital at the Feinberg School of Medicine, Northwestern University

Tell us more about your past. Did you always want to be a physician?
Actually, when I was a child I considered a career in engineering, because my parents were engineers.

What made you change your mind? What attracted you to medicine?
"Machines don't smile," as I say. Medicine gives you a profound level of satisfaction that no other career can provide. The grateful, sincere smile of a patient who survives after a close encounter with death; the tearful gratitude of a family whose child had been facing almost certain death—these cannot be replaced with anything. Nothing else can be so fulfilling, in my opinion.

How did you start your career in transplantation?
I started doing kidney transplants in my home country of Colombia, but I was particularly interested in liver, pancreas, living donor kidney, liver transplantation, and pediatric transplantation along with hepatobiliary surgery which represent a big unmet need. Unfortunately, there was no place to train for these types of surgeries in Colombia. One day, a Colombian surgeon working in the U.S. came to give a talk, so I approached him to ask about potential opportunities to work in the

U.S. I was disheartened to hear his tremendously negative perspective. He basically said that it would be impossible for me to train and practice in the U.S. because of the immigration issues, the language, and the competition would make it virtually impossible.

Similarly, when I was already a transplant surgeon in Colombia, I visited the U.S. to try and interview with different programs. One of my contacts, the Head of a Transplant Center in Florida, was a friend of my boss in Colombia.

When we spoke, he suggested that I work for him as a physician assistant for one year, before giving me the opportunity to start my fellowship. This was surprising, frustrating, and obviously not an option for me. I wanted to start my multivisceral abdominal transplant training. I was extremely focused on my dream.

What happened next?
I didn't speak any English, so I came to the Indiana University Bloomington, to learn. One day my classmates and I traveled to Chicago as tourists. However, because I had been dreaming about the possibility of visiting the Transplant Center, we drove by Northwestern University. As a tourist, wearing travel pants and with my camera bag — but my goals always front and center in my mind — I decided to walk in. Despite my broken English, I asked for the Chief of Transplantation who I knew was a past President of the American Society of Transplant Surgeons. The administrator was very kind to me. She asked for my CV, which I had saved on a floppy disk, and told me to wait an hour. (As a side note, for the kids of today who don't know what a floppy disk is, that is what we used to store data before CDs and flash drives.)

Did you manage to speak with him?
Yes. The wait paid off when Dr. Frank Stuart and Dr. Michael Abecassis came out and met me. I went straight to the point. I told them that I was interested in kidney, pancreas, liver transplantation, hepatobiliary surgery, living donor liver transplantation, and pediatric transplantation. I wanted to know if there was any opportunity for me at Northwestern. I realized that all this training implied three different fellowships and for that reason I clearly stated I was willing to invest whatever time was necessary if I had the opportunity. They were surprised for my clear and ambitious dream. My poor English didn't prevent us from having an hour a half long conversation. As opposed to the previous conversation with the specialist from Chicago who visited Colombia, Drs. Stuart and Abecassis gave me hope. They

said that I could do the three fellowships in multivisceral kidney, liver, pancreas transplantation, living donor liver transplantation, pediatric transplantation, and hepatobiliary surgery.

My question was whether there was an option for me to enroll in their program. They were kind enough to introduce me to a Chilean transplant fellow training with them who gave me a tour of the hospital and even allowed me to watch part of a surgery. After the tour, I went back to Drs. Stuart and Abecassis who told me that if I went through my title homologation and examination process, they could consider me. They did not say no. They gave me hope.

I went ahead and took the tests. I made probably every possible mistake in my USMLEs (homologation tests) but persevered and eventually succeeded. I applied to at least 20 transplant programs in the U.S. Some of them never got back to me. Others sent letters encouraging me to try again in a few, 10, or 20 years. I persisted and passed the USMLE testing and received the ECFMG certification. I completed all three fellowships at Northwestern University, (Northwestern Memorial Hospital and Lurie Children's Hospital) in 2006. My intention was to go back to my country. I felt bad about not returning to Colombia, leaving my people without that valuable resource, but creating a transplant program focused on Hispanics helped me to address my wish to help my people. The opportunity arose for me to stay in the United States, and I chose to take it because I recognized it was as an opportunity to help the Hispanic population here in the U.S. as there was NO Hispanic transplant program in the U.S. at that time. Ours was the first in the country. I saw the opportunity to give back to my people and we're still serving them.

What's your message for young Hispanics reading this book?
Be humble. Do not look for shortcuts. Persevere and spend the time to accomplish your goals. Make the effort. It can be done. Keep trying. Never give up.

If you have a clear dream, you must pursue it. You must knock on doors. Life will present you with many opportunities, but it's your responsibility to pursue them. The harder you work, the more likely you are to succeed. Luck favors those who work hard.

Tell us more about your current position and what you have accomplished.

I am an adult and pediatric transplant surgeon at Northwestern Memorial Hospital and Lurie Children's Hospital that ranked #1 in Illinois and top ten in the nation.

I am the director of the Hispanic Transplant Program. I am also the Surgical director of the Liver Transplant Program, director of the Living Donor Liver Transplant Program, and hepatobiliary surgery. I developed the Hispanic Kidney Transplant Program here at Northwestern Memorial Hospital in 2006 and the Hispanic Liver Transplant Program in 2010. I am currently director of the Hispanic Program, Surgical director of the Liver Transplant Program, and director of the Living Donor Liver Transplant Program, and hepatobiliary surgery.

We started the Northwestern Hispanic Transplant Program to solve an unmet need in the Hispanic population, not for research purposes. However, when we started to grow, we began considering doing research.

At the beginning, the need for a transplant program focused in Hispanic patients was questioned. However, we knew there was a disproportionate number of Hispanics receiving transplants compared with their representation in waiting lists. I started on my own and eventually a social worker joined me to help with education, brake cultural barriers, insurance/migratory issues, and other tasks. More importantly, she started with outreach programs, to answer questions, and help bring patients to the center. Over time, as the program grew, we brought more Spanish-speaking people. Now, we have almost 50 bilingual and bicultural transplant team members including three transplant surgeons, two hepatologists, one nephrologist, two transplant fellows, two social workers, several nurses, transplant coordinators, financial coordinators, assistants, one immunologist, and more. There are very few culturally competent and linguistically appropriate transplant services in the United States. The Hispanic Transplant Program at Northwestern Medicine is the first of its kind in the U.S.

Importantly, since the implementation of the Northwestern Hispanic Kidney Transplant Program, three major accomplishments deserve highlighting:

1.   access to transplant care (measured by addition to the kidney transplant waiting list) has increased by 91% among Hispanic Americans;
2.   the number of living donor kidney transplants in Hispanics has increased

by 74%, 9% of the transplants were among Hispanics before the Hispanic transplant program was implemented versus 25% of all transplants after;

3. the disparities in Hispanics decreased: the ratio of Hispanic to non-Hispanic White living donor kidney transplants has increased by 70%. Similar results have been seen in the Hispanic liver transplant program. Even though the Hispanic transplant program was a response to a need, it has also become an important research topic.

Because of our outcomes, [344, 345] we were able to receive our first National Institutes of Health (NIH) R01 grant. Our goal is to increase living kidney donation in Hispanics. We are implementing and evaluating the Hispanic transplant program in other centers across the country. We are teaching institutions like the Mayo Clinic (Arizona) and Baylor (Dallas, Texas) how to implement and evaluate culturally and linguistically competent and congruent transplant programs. The NIH R01 grant is a great accomplishment, because only 2% of transplant surgeons in the U.S. have an R01 grant.

I travel often to help other centers by giving talks and providing advice on how to develop this type of program. The program is currently used as a model for other institutions in the U.S. We hope that we have influenced the field to provide better education, better access to transplants, and better outcomes. Access is critical because many patients don't even know that this option exists.

The Northwestern Hispanic Transplant program has been a very satisfying endeavor for me because it not only allows us to help the Hispanic community and Hispanic physicians to get training and fulfill their dreams, but it has also helped me grow professionally.

Secondary to these efforts, I have received multiple awards/recognitions including:

- The Life Goes On award from the Illinois Secretary of State Jesse White (2008) for promoting organ donation and transplantation among Hispanics.

- Crain's Chicago Business' Top 40 under 40 (2009) for developing the Hispanic transplant program, at Northwestern Memorial Hospital at the efforts to increase organ donation and transplantation in the Hispanic community.

- The Heroes for Hope Real-life Llifesavers award (2013) from Gift of Hope, Organ and Tissue Donor Network, Organ procurement organization (OPO).

-The Gift of Life Award from the National Kidney Foundation of Illinois (2016) for developing a bilingual and culturally sensitive website (Informate.com) to increase knowledge about living kidney donation and transplantation among Latino/Hispanic communities.

- I have also become the only Hispanic Board member of influential organizations in organ donation and transplantation including Gift of hope (OPO) and National Kidney foundation of Illinois and a member of the OPTN/ UNOS affairs committee. I was also the inaugural Chair of the American Society of Transplant Surgeons Diversity issue committee.

What's the most rewarding aspect of your role?
I think that the most rewarding is to be an instrument of hope, giving a new option of life to many people who would die without a transplant. I remember a liver transplant patient spent 17 minutes in cardiac arrest (clinically death) during surgery, and who survived and is still enjoying life with her family. To see them walk out of the hospital gives you a feeling of fulfillment and accomplishment that cannot be compared.

Another rewarding aspect is the opportunity to help other Hispanics who dream about practicing in the U.S. My goal has been to give hope as opposed to what I heard when I was looking for opportunities. I have mentored several surgeons, residents, undergraduate, and high school students at Northwestern. Several fellows have come as observers and felt the motivation. We have helped open doors to other Hispanic surgeons. We have trained at least ten of them—one U.S. born, the rest trained in Latin America (Colombia, Mexico, Venezuela, Argentina, Chile and Brazil).

In line with this wonderful story, do you have an author or a quote from a favorite author that you think about often?
Yes. My favorite quote is from St. Francis of Assisi: "Start by doing what's necessary; then do what's possible; and suddenly you are doing the impossible."

LATANYA BENJAMIN

Latanya Benjamin, MD, FAAD is double board certified pediatric dermatologist, former Professor at Stanford University and renowned Pediatric Dermatologic Surgeon.

When and how did you become interested in Medicine?
At an early age, I knew I wanted to be either a doctor or a teacher. My earliest memory is of my mother bringing me a book she found at the library with information on basic facts about becoming a doctor.

I became the first generation of my family to migrate to this country and the first doctor in my family. Like many, my parents supported me and instilled the value of studying and working hard in school to get good grades. But with no other true example or guidance at home to become a doctor, I (we) just kinda figured it out.

Can you tell us about a life-changing moment related to your choice of career?
I knew I was going to be a pediatrician since the age of 15. By my senior year of medical school I was deliberating over which specialty in pediatrics would be the best fit. Up until this point, I had no exposure to dermatology in medical school (very late in the game).

It was during the time of I was applying for a residency that I attended a Friday afternoon clinic in pediatric dermatology and everything clicked! I immediately knew this was my career choice. It encompassed everything I loved—continuity of care, acute care, chronic care, procedural care. I now found a career path that blended my two greatest passions, taking care of children (pediatrics) and dermatology.

That very evening I called my parents because I was just about to match in a categorical pediatric residency and I told my parents that they won't understand what I am going to do but that I found my career and that I would somehow figure out how I would accomplish it and that we would be in for a long ride.

What are your key responsibilities in your present role and how did you arrive at this position?
My key responsibility is to provide the best cutting-edge dermatologic care for children. I am a trusted medical expert and therefore hold additional roles that help to shape the future of my specialty and young physicians in training. I enjoy teaching students, and as an Associate Professor, have taught student doctors at every level of training. I hold executive officer/board of director positions with national and local dermatology societies and sit at the table for multiple medical advisory boards. I have a heart for advocacy and volunteerism and enjoy giving back to communities.

What is the most fulfilling aspect of your current role?
Taking care of children and supporting others to succeed in their career aspiration in medicine.

What are you most proud of in your personal and professional journey?
Teaching as a Professor at Stanford University, publishing the first-ever medical textbook devoted to pediatric dermatology surgery and other procedures for children, and giving birth to my daughter.

What are your most important personal and professional values?
To always remain ethical. Honesty, integrity, professionalism, and having a hard-work ethic follows closely. Professionally, it also means always doing what is best for the patient first, listening to and valuing the opinions and concerns of their parents. Personally, I feel proud of taking the high road and pursuing excellence in everything I do.

What is the main lesson you have learned since starting your career in medicine?
Perseverance will serve you! The journey is longer and harder than you could ever imagine. Remain fluid and adapt. That will enable you to benefit and grow from those unexpected detours in your career and surprises of life. With time, it's beautiful to discover who you are and who you are not.

If you could go back in time and do something different, what would that be?
I would be bold, ask questions and speak up. I would avoid doing the journey alone;

I would study with peers, seek support and identify a mentor sooner.

How do you define success?
Success looks different for everyone. For me, it is creating the life that you desire and deserve to have, with your heart in the right place, wanting good for others as well.

Did you have a mentor? Can you tell us how he or she helped you get to where you are?
During an undergraduate year at the University of Florida, I was a member of the Hispanic club. I was paired with a mentor I will never forget, Dr. Lourdes Corman. She was the first female mentor I had in college who helped guide me while I was selecting which medical schools to apply to. She told me about various medical schools I never even knew about, one of which ended up being the medical school I would later earn my medical degree from.

What have you received in terms of advice and mentorship that has pushed you to where you are today?
During my training at Northwestern, my fellowship director Dr. Anthony Mancini gave me the best advice. He said, "Why put off until tomorrow what you can do today?" This truly helped me through a period of procrastination when I felt overwhelmed, and helps me remain productive to this very day.

Based on your experience, what is the main advantage of a career in medicine? Do you see it as a key area of opportunity for Hispanics?
Medicine affords me the ability to serve humanity by offering my knowledge, compassion and care during difficult times and sometimes critical moments in a patient's life. Even the ability to comfort and reassure goes a long way as a specialist in medicine. In a clinic setting, whether you see one, four or eight persons in an hour, that's the bare minimum of how many lives and families and communities you are impacting. And for some, you get to become a part of that person's story. To me that is the main advantage of a career in medicine.

Absolutely, Hispanics are the fastest growing population in the U.S., outpacing the number of physicians entering medicine Therefore, there is a great need and it is a key area of opportunity for this population to be served by another who understands the Hispanic family and culture. You become a role model to various generations just by having them see a Hispanic doctor walking through the door.

Why did you decide to become involved in developing new Hispanic talent in medicine? How has this enriched your own trajectory?
There is a great need for diversity in medicine, especially in the field of dermatology. I am very active as a mentor in developing new Hispanic talent in medicine. I am devoted to helping young students and trainees, especially ethnic women, know that they can rise to new heights given their capabilities, compassion and intellect. I see them all as competent individuals deserving to be in the role that they want to be in. This reminds me how far I've come and how far we have yet to go. It is important to me to give back what I've been given.

What steps do we need to take to address the shortage of Hispanic physicians in the U.S.? Why is it important to help increase Latino representation in medicine?
I believe two things are greatly needed. First, scholarship programs for underrepresented minorities will make a huge impact. Often times, the barrier is a matter of finance. Most people don't realize how much money is required to fund a career in medicine. The basic includes medical school loans, the cost to take multiple board and other exams, the monies needed to apply to and interview at multiple training programs across the country, cost to be credentialed, licensed and verified multiple times throughout ones career, pay dues, and the cost associated to take CME courses and attend medical conferences to maintain a medical license.

The second would be effective mentoring programs to give Hispanics early exposure to the field of medicine, as well as providing exposure beyond primary care to the various subspecialties within medicine, which tend to be more lucrative. Mentors who serve as role models will offer guidance as to how it is done at different stages in along the career path. There is a lot of talent among Latinos and they need our help in receiving the advantages needed to become competent doctors who are culturally sensitive.

If you had unlimited resources, what action would you prioritize to help young Hispanics living in the U.S. who are interested in pursuing careers in medicine?
I would provide financial assistance and develop active, effective mentorship programs in every school throughout the country to offer students early exposure to different fields of medicine. Middle and high school students would first get

shadowing opportunities and college students would be partnered with a practicing Hispanic physicians.

What advice do you have for others who want to follow your path?
Go for it! It takes grit to follow this path and acquire the dream, so don't be afraid to work hard and believe in delayed gratification.

Do you have an author or a quote from a favorite author that you think of often?
"The journey of a thousand miles begins with a single step."- Lao Tzu

If you were giving a speech at a high school or medical school commencement, what advice would you give?
Choose medicine for yourself. Be sure it is truly your passion and purpose and not the desire of your parents or family or because you envision it will make you rich. It takes a long time, lots of dedication and hard work and only you get to walk the walk. If it's for you, then grab every chance for exposure....see as much, do as much, be as much, give as much as you can possibly can. This is the philosophy I live by.

What book(s) would you recommend to young Hispanic students interested in a career in medicine?
Your textbooks. Study, study hard. The more basic medicine you learn, no matter what field you ultimately choose, the better a doctor you will be.

Any parting words of wisdom?
Being a minority in medicine is an honor and a privilege. I am a person of mixed ethnicities. I feel this deeper cultural understanding makes me more relatable to the families in which I serve. Be proud of your unique self! Your existence is guaranteed to serve someone else as a role model in medicine.

MARIETTA VASQUEZ

Marietta Vázquez, M.D. is a Professor of Pediatrics at the Yale University School of Medicine.

She is an Infectious Diseases specialist, Vice-Chair of Diversity Equity and Inclusion, and Director of the Yale Children's Hispanic Clinic.

Dr. Vázquez graduated Cum Laude from Yale University School of Medicine and has been the recipient of the Morris Y. Krosnick Award, the Robert Wood Johnson Foundation Minority Medical Faculty Development Award, the May Gailani Junior Faculty Award, the Charles C. Shephard Science Award and the Physician Traiblazer Award.

Tell us about your early life and how you become interested in Medicine?
I'm the daughter of Cuban parents who emigrated in the early 1960s, when the Castro regime took over. They married and settled in Puerto Rico, where I was born and raised. My story begins on the sunny streets where my mind slowly but surely built up a dream: becoming a doctor.

My studies have taken me back and forth between Puerto Rico and the United States. I completed high school in Puerto Rico and attended college in the United States at Yale University. I went back to my country for medical school at the University of Puerto Rico School of Medicine,. During medical school, I became interested in the field of pediatric infectious diseases, but since there are no fellowship programs in Puerto Rico, I knew I had to return to the United States for subspecialty training. I understood early of the importance of self-motivation and seeking opportunities myself.

During my years as a medical student was the beginning of the AIDS epidemic, I became very enthralled by this new virus that was affecting so many children in Puerto Rico for which we knew very little about; there was so much more to know about it, and I became interested in engaging in research as a means to find out more. AIDS Research at that time was not a priority at the University of Puerto Rico; there were little opportunities for medical students, or even people to talk to about it. I was very interested in what was happening with the AIDS virus, mostly having to do with illness in children. The atmosphere in the medical world was fascinating as if science was at a turning point-- I craved to learn, to help, to be a part of something greater than myself. In our youth, isn't that what we are all hungry for?

Knowing the Centers for Disease and Control (CDC) was the epicenter of clinical research in pediatric AIDS, I started looking at names of researchers and leaders at CDC. I came across a Hispanic name. I asked around in my medical school and they told me this person was from Puerto Rico, just like me! I wrote him a long, long, letter about who I was and what I wanted to do in the future, and why he should help me find a summer internship at CDC. I poured my entire soul in that letter. Then I sat and waited, and waited, and waited. Back then there was no email, everything was slower, and people were harder to reach. But, nothing is impossible. I ended up getting that summer research internship at CDC cementing my lifelong interest in a career in infectious diseases research.

After medical school I returned to the United States, specifically to Yale, and completed pediatric residency training. At the time, I was the only Hispanic in the Yale pediatrics program. I started in that program in 1994 and it wasn't until 2017 that another Puerto Rican joined it.

Can share a life-changing moment in your career?
When I think of a turning point in my career I think back to a very simple interaction—one that showed me how I, as a doctor, could connect with the Latino community and make a difference although I was so far away from home In the first few months after I came to the U.S., I took care of a little girl. Her parents were farm workers and she had leukemia. Although I was a pediatric resident back then, I helped the family understand the disease, its treatment and became an advocate for her.

At Yale, forty percent of the patients who shared a ZIP code with the New Haven Hospital, which is the city where Yale is located, came from households listing Spanish as their primary language. This meant that a huge proportion of our patients were Hispanic. During my residency I often felt as if there were two very different worlds: the diverse community we served and Yale, a prestigious, academic ivory tower. Often I felt as if I stood alone on a bridge, right between two very different worlds that I was connected to, but not quite a part of. It took time, but eventually I learned how this shaped my role as someone who serves by bridging differences. Many of the patients I took care of were Hispanic, I always saw it as a benefit to me, as I learned so much from them; it wasn't until a few years later that I started understanding the bi-directionality of the relationship, in terms of its benefit to the community and dreamt of one day having a clinic just for Hispanic patients

Over the last 25 years of my career as a physician-scientist continued to develop. I gained expertise in patient care, developed a research career in the field of vaccines, became involved in global medicine and in medical education and had the fortune to be able to mentor others. I grew a lot professionally. But this dream was something that was always in the back of my mind. I spent hours on end thinking about it, talking it through with colleagues, friends and even my patients.

Finally, eight years ago I started a Hispanic clinic for children and their families at Yale. It felt like the right time—the proportion of Hispanics in the community had increased and over the years there was more connection between the institution and the community.

The clinic is called Y-CHiC—an acronym for the Yale-Clinic for Hispanic Children or Yale—(Clínica Hispana para Chicos); it provides medical care that is language and culturally- competent. About 90-95% of the patients at Y-CHiC are undocumented immigrants from all over Latin-America. At Y-CHiCe've we celebrate culture, including food and music with the purpose of bonding patients together and making them feel safe and comfortable. If people come in and they hear their music, and taste their food and hear their doctor speak their language, it just gives them a sense of belonging and trust. That is one of the things I'm most proud of. Many of our providers are not Hispanic, but through that space they not only learn more about medicine, but about what it means to be Hispanic—about culture and language competence which, in addition to warming our patients' hearts, actually improves our service.

I believe that the work we do at our clinic is a great example of the small steps we can take in the right direction. We have proven that you don't need an entire team of fifty exclusively Hispanic professionals, but that one person can make the difference.

When comparing our patients at Y-CHiC with those of the traditional Yale clinic, our patients are less likely to miss their appointments, more likely to feel that their doctor knows their child, and that they know their doctor, more likely to do something as simple as remembering their doctor's name. Data has shown that if you share language, if you share background, if you share similar beliefs, this leads to better understanding between patient and doctor. In more practical terms, understanding the language and addressing the cultural aspects of social determinants of health, will contribute to achieving better outcomes.

There's a saying about how you can't be what you don't see. You can tell young Latino kids that they are going to be President of the United States, but if they have never seen a Hispanic President of the United States, they're not going to genuinely believe that they can. I think this applies to patients. When they go to into a medical center, and they see somebody like them, more trust is developed.

Eventually Hispanics will become the largest population of the United States, but we're not going to be able to have a native speaker for every Hispanic patient. And that is far from goal. I'll always remember receiving at the clinic patients from Guatemala who spoke dialects that I don't understand. Should they have a doctor that is exclusively for them? Ideally, maybe. But realistically, what they deserve, what we all deserve, in my opinion, are capable professionals, educated in cultural competence. I believe it's our duty to not only enhance and diversify our medical field, but also to educate, and that's one of my goals as vice chair of diversity, equity and inclusion in my department: to teach cultural competence and help with language competence. I dream of this goal becoming a widespread rule. So that we all understand each other better.

I always compare it with flu vaccines. When I was a trainee we always knew that everybody should get an influenza vaccine. If you're a health care provider and you don't get flu vaccine, it can be detrimental to your patients. But it wasn't until recently that getting the flu vaccine became mandatory. Well, I see diversity training, and cultural competence and all of these things about equity, and inclusion, very similarly to that. This type of education should be mandatory. When hospitals and departments are cited for lack of diversity, then they take action. However, is it the right thing to be reactive rather than proactive? No.

In summary, we have a community that needs and deserves doctors they can relate to. Along with a very caring team, we have visited community fairs, local schools, and as many events as we can organize. In these events, we present learning activities in the hope of inspiring our youth to follow their dreams, and hopefully pursue a career in the medical field. Some activities include showing them how to listen to somebody's heart, how to do deep tendon reflexes, things that are very, very simple but that will inspire kids greatly. With experience I've learned that sometimes the most I can contribute is to simply say, "I'm a doctor, I speak your language, I come from the same country that your parents came from and let me tell you how I got to where I am now."

However, I've also learned that I can't do this alone. To organize these events, even the smallest one, I need at least a team of twenty. I guarantee that a single person can make a difference, but what if our first task is to inspire others, inspire our peers? The things that we could achieve together are endless.

When you ask me about what I would do if I had unlimited resources, I can only think of education. I think that a big part of why young Hispanics in our school systems do not get the help that they need is lack of awareness. It is that sometimes the teachers don't understand the realities of the student's parents and the difficulties they go through. They don't understand that two years ago, maybe their parents were not leaving the house, maybe their parents were very wary of going outside, because they thought that they were going to get deported. Maybe the teachers don't understand that the rate of depression and suicide in our country is the highest among young Hispanic females. Maybe they don't understand that students who are not U.S. citizens only have access to an education through high school. And what happens after that? If you're a young person who got straight A's and performed very well academically, you're going to see your peers go off to college, but you can't go. You would need to pay not only full tuition, but you may even need to pay the international rate because you're not a United States citizen.

So my answer would be education for everybody. If I had unlimited resources, I would start by saying that health care and education should be a right and not a privilege and that everybody should have access not only a primary and secondary education, but also a college education. I think that would go a long way. It's very hard when you don't have the money, when your parents don't speak the language, when you don't have the mentor, and on top of that, you don't even have access to student loans.

Mentors are also instrumental. I can credit part of my academic success to valuable mentorship. One of my mentors, perhaps the most notable in my entire career, is an older white man. Although not my age, not my race, not my gender, nor my ethnicity, this person has impacted my career significantly and exemplified how I approach mentoring others.

Some of my mentees over the years have been young people who researching potential mentors and found my "Hispanic" name and reached out to me--just like I did so many years ago. Having motivation and resilience has paid off. Now it's my turn to encourage other dreamers out there to keep going, to fight for their dreams, to take every opportunity they can get, be the best they can be, and do something with their lives to help others and give back.

In the end, we need to understand where we come from, what our values are, seeking growth opportunities and being brave to pursue one's dreams.

NINA RAMIREZ

Dr. Ramirez, M.D., FAAAAI, FCCP is a practicing Allergist & Immunologist in Pembroke Pines, FL.

Dr. Ramirez graduated from Weill Cornell Medical College in 1978 and has been in practice for 41 years.

She currently practices at Asthma and Allergy Associates of Florida and is Past President of the Florida Allergy Asthma and Immunology Society

I was born and raised on the Island of Manhattan, New York City. My life's journey began at an Ivy League institution, Columbia Presbyterian's Babies Hospital, directly across the street from my parent's bodega in upper Manhattan. Born to two wonderfully supportive parents from the Island of Puerto Rico I was blessed with their work ethic, spirit and determination to succeed when opportunities presented themselves. Without their love and belief in me I would not be sharing this narrative with you today. No one could have ever imagined that by the age of 25, I would be the recipient of an MD degree from another world-class Ivy League institution, Weill-Cornell College of Medicine. Decades later my journey continues.

I attended one of the specialized high schools in New York City known then as the High School of Music and Art. Like many of my fellow classmates furthering music studies at a conservatory seemed inevitable. Remarkably, as a violinist, my interest in the sciences began with high school biology. I never attended a conservatory after high school. Eventually and by default, I thought about becoming a teacher. It was during my sophomore year in college that my chemistry professor encouraged me to think about a career in medicine. He apparently saw something special in me that I did not see in myself and challenged me to 'do my homework' before making any decisions about the future.

So, in the summer between my sophomore and junior years at Fordham University I volunteered in the evenings at Columbia Presbyterian Hospital. I was designated as a floater to go where I was needed. One evening, I was assigned to the ER and asked to help a woman surgeon who needed assistance in repairing a large laceration on the arm of a teenager. These were the days before privacy statutes would have prevented this act of fate. The ER was short staffed. I remember the surgeon asking if the sight of blood bothered me. I thought about my father who was also a butcher at the bodega. He often had blood on his white apron from cutting meat. I just smiled to myself and responded with a confident no. The next thing I knew I was asked to wash my hands and dress with a gown, cap, gloves and mask. For the next 2 hours I sat on a stool holding retractors for the surgeon. I was never the same after that evening. I returned in the fall of my junior year to Fordham University and declared myself a pre-med major. I am forever grateful for my professor's encouragement.

From that moment forward my destiny became more apparent. I developed a keen sense of tunnel vision staying focused despite my naivete about the challenges that lie ahead. The first 2 years of medical school required tremendous effort to comprehend the vast quantity of brand-new subject matter related to the basic sciences. I had challenges, struggles, and setbacks along the way. But by the third year I felt a light bulb had gone off in my head and things began to fall into place. Like the 'rise of the phoenix' I began to soar and develop a greater focus on my future path.

Now years later, I get to make a difference in someone's life. As a physician my interest is caring for infants, children and adults with allergic diseases including severe persistent asthma. Because of the tremendous advancements in our understanding of these disease states, we can offer those who suffer relief and continued hope. It is enormously rewarding to watch a person's suffering come to an end.

Ironically, I became a teacher after all. I teach patients about their disease and treatment options; I educate the other doctors about long-term management strategies and I share this good news when mentoring medical students and residents in training.

I am currently a Fellowship Trained and Board-Certified consultant in Adult and Pediatric Allergy-Immunology and Pediatric Pulmonology. After completing a residency in Pediatrics at the Mount Sinai Hospital in New York City I pursued additional training as a Pulmonologist at both Mount Sinai and Children's Hospital National Medical Center in Washington, D.C. The following 15 years my career focused on caring for infants, children, and young adults with a variety of respiratory diseases.

In the year 2000, during my twenty second post graduate year from medical school, I had the opportunity to return to additional Fellowship training in the field of Allergy and Immunology at the University of South Florida. I sat for and passed the Board Certification examination in Allergy-Immunology in 2014, twenty years after my initial certification as a Pediatric Pulmonologist.

In 2018 I became the first Latina, 4th woman, and 69th President of the Florida Allergy, Asthma, and Immunology Society.

Throughout my journey I have been gifted with wonderful professors and mentors who have encouraged me along the way. I would not be where I am today were it not for them. Some of my greatest teachers have also been the patients I have cared for over the years. They have taught me how to be a better listener and a more compassionate physician. Their well-being motivates me to learn more. They are a source of great inspiration.

On a personal note, I could not be prouder of my daughter, Natalie. As an actor and educator, I am awestruck by her use of the time, talent, and treasures she has been given to foster tremendous growth and wisdom in her students. She has often served as my coach when preparing for public speaking engagements. Natalie brings out the best in me.

A career in medicine is a universal calling. As universal citizens, our job as physicians is to lift the burden of our fellow man regardless of their identity or social status. With the demographics of the United States rapidly shifting many of our patients are Hispanics and naturally gravitate towards and seek physicians with whom they share a common bond. This is indeed a privilege and a challenge to impart our knowledge in a meaningful way. While many are bilingual, there is no doubt some prefer to narrate their story in Spanish. What they have to say is important and they prefer to say it in Spanish!

I have been asked what I would do with access to limitless resources to encourage students like yourselves. This was not a difficult task. I would start a future doctor's club at the elementary, middle school and high school levels in major metropolitan cities with a large Latino presence. This road show-and-tell would bring Hispanic physicians to your auditoriums throughout the United States talking about a career in medicine. The t-shirts would read, "Si se puede! Yes you can!" The dream starts early. The path is long, but worth every challenging bit of it!

My advice to those seeking a similar path is to have patience, fortitude, aptitude and a whole lot of attitude. There will be those who doubt your sincerity and capability. There were those who doubted mine.

From Felix Marti-Ibanez's book To Be A Doctor these words best summarize the journey. 'To be a doctor is, in other words, to be a whole person, a good person, who fulfills his or her task as a scientist with professional quality and integrity; as a human being with a kind heart and high ideals; and as a member of society, with honesty and efficiency...you are embarking on a noble career in which there is no room for amateurs or dilettanti, a career in which we must all aspire to be masters of whatever we undertake...'.

This book was given to me upon graduation from medical school in 1978. The dedication read, 'To Nina, Run a good race and fight a good battle and may love, peace, and fulfillment be yours through medicine'.

Now is your time to run a good race and fight the noble battle.
Society needs you!

CONCLUDING REMARKS

The first steps toward medical school

"If you have faith even as tiny as a mustard seed,
all things are possible."
- Aida Giachello, Ph.D. Latino Health Activist

ANA MARIA
IS GOING TO
COLLEGE

I first met Ana Maria online more than two years ago.

When I spoke with her recently to let her know that the book was almost ready, I was happy to hear that she's made so much progress.

"Did you know that the government has a program that helps you pay for your med school applications?" Ana Maria asked me.

"No. I didn't know!"

"I didn't know either, but I did some research and found out that they can pay for all ten of my applications!

"I work hard to be able to go to school. My parents are still struggling. Nothing has changed at home, but I did some volunteer EMS work for a while and started tutoring kids in my neighborhood who come from immigrant families and don't speak English well yet. It's not like I make a lot of money doing that because these families are poor, but I made enough to pay for part of my EMT training, and it feels good to help these kids anyway!

"I have a plan now. I just started working as an EMT every weekend and I'm trying to save as much as I can. Because I'll have to keep working, I know that it will take me longer to graduate than people with more resources, but I'm ok with that.

"Also, I started talking to everyone about my dream and I just met a doctor at the cafe where I go do my homework…" she paused, "because of the free internet," she whispered," and he said that he'll try to see if he can let me come to the hospital to shadow one of the residents."

"Wow! I'm so happy to hear that Ana Maria. It sounds like you're doing really well."

"Yes! I'm so glad I didn't let that counselor discourage me, and thank you for telling my story in your book. I just want to take the opportunity to tell other young people like me to not give up. It's hard, you know. I work hard, and sometimes all I eat is one sandwich the entire day! But it's worth it. I really want to give back. I hope that one day I will be able to help patients who don't speak English, like my mom and dad. I don't want other parents to go through what they have experienced with my sister."

"On the contrary," I said, "thank you for inspiring me. I think we can both encourage everyone reading this book to share at least one thing they learned from it—maybe your story, Ana Maria, or the story of one of the doctors I interviewed, or perhaps one of the pieces of information from the data sections. We all need to know our community better. Knowledge is power.

"Is there anything else you want to tell other students like you?"

"Just one thing: Don't give up and don't let anybody ever tell you that you can't achieve your dream."

There is no simple answer to the question "Why do we need more Hispanic physicians and scientists in the U.S.?" In their article, "Disparities In Human Resources: Addressing The Lack Of Diversity In The Health Professions," [120] Grumbach and Mendoza make the case for increasing diversity in the health professions. There is **a civil rights case**, based on the recognition of the country's history of segregation and inequality that justifies the need for policies such as affirmative action; **a business case**, based on improved customer service and decreased long-term cost that results when patients do not need to keep coming back to receive healthcare; **an educational case**, supported by the known benefits to individuals who are educated among a diverse school population; and **a public health case**, supported by research demonstrating that patients treated by racially concordant physicians or by physicians who are linguistically and culturally competent are more satisfied with the clinical encounter and have better outcomes. One of the key objectives of this book is to support the public health case for diversity in medicine.

Like other minorities, Hispanics receive lower quality healthcare than Whites. The data presented throughout this book tell a compelling story of inequality in which fewer Hispanics pursue careers in medicine, not because of lack of interest or ability, but because of lack of opportunity that begins early in life. However, the numbers also tell us that Hispanics are going to school in record numbers and that those who make it to college do as well as students of other races. In addition, the numbers show us that Hispanic physicians care for a larger percentage of Hispanic patients, and that more Hispanic patients choose to see Hispanic physicians and rate their interactions with those doctors higher. Thus, the numbers demonstrate the importance of culturally and linguistically competent health care.

Enormous efforts have been made by both public and private organizations to provide health care providers with cultural competence training. However, standardized training and outcome measures are not yet broadly in place. Cultural competence programs are heterogeneous, ranging from one-hour webinars or seminars to several weeks of either online or in-person training. I want to stress my belief that cultural and linguistic competence training is absolutely critical. However, when asked about the benefits of these different training modalities, many physicians agree that a few hours of education cannot possibly prepare a healthcare provider to deal with the tremendous diversity of their patient population. Standardized programs with appropriate measures to track patient outcomes after the intervention are what is needed.

Linguistic competence is the linguistic knowledge possessed by native speakers of a language. With such a disparity in the number of Spanish-speaking physicians compared to their English-speaking colleagues, providing linguistically appropriate care is even more difficult. In addition, effective communication is not only about language proficiency but about the ability to appreciate the culture relative to the spoken language. This ranges from understanding the ingredients of a traditional dish that could have caused a symptom, to being familiar with the names of frequently used natural remedies; from knowing what words or phrases to use to help a patient cope with a difficult diagnosis, to knowing how to explain instructions related to medications. Even the most culturally competent and compassionate physician could have difficulties managing a patient who does not speak his/her language. Interpreters help, but they are not always readily available, particularly in emergency situations, in health care centers with a large volume of patients, in remote locations, and when specific needs arise, such as interpreting for pediatric or elderly populations. [346] The current situation is obviously exceptional, but the COVID-19 pandemic is demonstrating the tremendous impact of a public health disaster on disadvantaged individuals, including those with low English proficiency in situations of high demand.

Increasing the number of Hispanics in health professions will require significant changes at many levels and will take years. This book is not about policy or political intervention. Other great works have been published recently on those topics.[181] Instead, as shown by the stories of the Hispanic doctors in Section Four of this book, success is possible at the individual level with effort and perseverance.

"Experience has taught me that you cannot value dreams according to the odds of their coming true. Their real value is in stirring within us the will to aspire."

−Sonya Sotomayor

The key for some students may be in the acceptance, by themselves and by our society as a whole, that the "traditional" path to medical school does not apply to many 21st century students, particularly those exposed to risk factors such as those described in this book.

This leads to the idea proposed by numerous authors and organizations of a **post-traditional student**, [347-349] an individual who may take numerous paths to medical school. The term defines a heterogeneous group of individuals: from high school graduates and high school dropouts, to students with limited English language skills; from millennials who feel the need to customize their learning experiences, to young adults already in the workforce who may be single parents, or trying to make a career change, or trying resume a career that was put on hold for financial reasons. These students may not fit the traditional educational timeline and often need help meeting the requirements for entry, navigating the system, obtaining financial aid, understanding career options, while earning wages to support themselves and their families.

The organization Excelencia in Education has proposed using a Latino lens to reimagine the post-traditional student's educational journey, in a way similar to the way our protagonist, Ana Maria has done. Their new student profile describes a student who may not be ready for college but is ready to take academic prep courses; a student who could enroll at a community college, or attend college part-time. It also includes someone who already has a job or could enter the workforce to save money to help with college tuition, or could work a significant portion of each week and take longer to complete a degree; a student who could live off-campus with family members or roommates and make choices according to cost and location.

In line with the post-traditional student persona, many Hispanics that I spoke with while writing this book told me that they knew they wanted to become doctors but did not know where to start. Some had been out of school and working for a while because they needed to support their families. Others had not yet finished high school and did not know where to find information about the cost of medical school, the application process, etc. For this reason, in addition to the online resources shared throughout the book, I wanted to end it by humbly offering a starting point that I shared with several students I met throughout this journey and was considered helpful. I see a three-step process for both a traditional and post-traditional student's path to medical school. Needless to say, this is an oversimplification, but use it as a way to organize your journey. Think of each of the three steps as an empty bucket that you need to fill in with information until you have a plan in place.

The first three steps toward medical school

1. Decide if medical school is right for you.

Whether you are making this decision because of a life-changing event like Ana Maria's experience with her sister, or because you truly believe that helping others is at the core of who you are, there is no doubt that medicine as a career requires effort and sacrifice.

> *The indispensable first step to getting the things you want out of life is this: decide what you want.*
> — *Ben Stein*

Think about it carefully before deciding whether medical school is right for you. Talk to your family and friends, talk to doctors and medical school students in your community who can share their stories. Volunteer at your local hospital and engage in healthcare-related activities even if only online in these times of social distancing, so you gain a clear understanding of the road ahead. Seek help from advisors and use online resources such as the ones included throughout this book. Importantly, once you have made your decision, do not let anybody discourage you. If I had listened to all the people who told me that achieving this career would take too long and be too difficult, I would not be where I am. Find a mentor. Someone who encourages you and helps you set ambitious yet realistic goals.

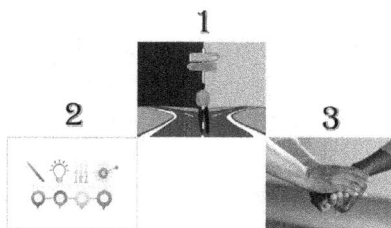

Where to start? 1. Decide 2. Plan 3. Keep the end in mind

FIGURE 54. A THREE-STEP PLAN TOWARDS MEDICAL SCHOOL

Once you have made the decision to go to medical school, you need an action plan. Conduct as much research as you can, use the resources provided in this book and share additional resources with others. Talk to people who are

"A goal without a plan is just a wish."

- Antoine de Saint-Exupéry

already in medical school and who can share their experiences. Talk to your primary care physician or find a doctor in your community who may be willing to spend a few minutes discussing his or her career path with you. Go to trustworthy blogs and websites, such as the AAMC and the AMA, and put together a plan based on the amount of time and money it would take for you in your specific circumstances to get ready to apply to medical school. The AAMC offers great information on every aspect of the journey to medical school and beyond. Ask yourself questions like "Am I prepared for the tests?" If your answer is "No," find free resources to help you study or determine how much a prep course would cost and whether they offer financial aid. Do not assume that because prep courses are expensive you have no access to them. There are options for test preparation and there are even summer programs that are free. I have included some links in this book, but ask med school students for more information. They may even be willing to help you and share their materials with you. Also, consider apps and YouTube videos uploaded by medical schools and nonprofit organizations that address the application and admission process, as well as test preparation.

I cannot overemphasize the importance of a plan of action. People from all walks of life who are successful will tell you that you cannot succeed without a plan. Conduct extensive research on the types of schools that you could apply to, the cost of the application and tuition, the opportunities for financial support, the length of time that it would take you to complete your training if you were still working part-time, etc. Set up timelines and goals, keeping in mind that your goals need to be SMART. [350-352]

- **S**pecific — Identify your goal clearly
- **M**easurable — How will you measure progress and accomplishment?
- **A**ttainable — The goal should have at least 50% chance of success.
- **R**elevant — The goal must be important and relevant to you.
- **T**ime-bound — You must commit to a specific time frame.

3. Begin with the end in mind

The process will be arduous and it may take a long time, especially if you have a job or other responsibilities, but always keep in mind what the goal is: to help others by providing linguistic and culturally competent care that improves people's lives. Regularly reminding yourself of your end goal will help you stay focused and strong throughout the process. Finally, look at yourself in the mirror like the girl on the cover of this book and use the mantra "Yes, I can!"

I wish you the best.

"To begin with the end in mind means to start with a clear understanding of your destination. It means to know where you're going so that you better understand where you are now and so that the steps you take are always in the right direction."

- Stephen R. Covey

Be a dream sower

First THINK

Second BELIEVE

Third DREAM

And finally, DARE

- Walt Disney

APPENDIX

GLOSSARY

Access – the ability to use needed health services by a patient or population in terms of the following: health services delivery system characteristics such as availability, organization, and financing of services; characteristics of the population such as demographics, income, care-seeking behavior; and whether or not the care sought adequately met the individual or group's basic medical needs.

Adjusted Cohort Graduation Rate (ACGR) – first collected for 2010-11, the ACGR is a graduation rate measure of the percentage of U.S. public high school students who graduate on time. To calculate the ACGR, states divide the number of those who graduate, by the number of students from an adjusted cohort for the graduating class. The states identify the "cohort" of first-time 9th graders in a particular school year, and adjust this number by adding any students who transfer into the cohort after 9th grade and subtracting any students who transfer out, immigrate to another country, or pass away. The ACGR is the percentage of the students in this cohort who graduate within four years. States calculate the ACGR for individual schools and districts and for the state as a whole using detailed data that track each student over time. In many states, these student-level records have become available at a state level only in recent years. As an example, the ACGR formula for 2012-13 was calculated like this:

Number of cohort members who earned a regular high school diploma by the end of the 2012- 13 school year

---

Number of first time 9th graders in fall 2009 (starting cohort) plus students who transferred in, minus students who transferred out, emigrated, or died during school years 2009-10, 2010-11, 2011-12, and 2012-13

Confounding factor – a component of a research study that has a strong relationship with one of the variables, making it impossible to separate how much of the observed effect was due to the intervention and how much was due to the confounding factor.

Cultural Competence – refers to the knowledge, interpersonal skills, behaviors, attitudes, and policies that allow health professions educators and practitioners to understand, appreciate, and respect cultural differences and similarities in cross-cultural situations. Cultural competency acknowledges these variances in customs, values, beliefs, and communication patterns by incorporating these variables in the assessment and treatment of individuals and in the training of all health professionals. The goal is to provide information and services in the language and educational and cultural context most appropriate for the individuals you serve.

Demonym (from Greek, dêmos, "people, tribe" and ónoma, "name") – identifies residents or natives of a particular place and is usually derived from the name of the place. For example, American, Peruvian, Ecuadorian. The word demonym does not take into account ethnicity. For instance, an Ecuadorian may be a resident of Ecuador belonging to any ethnic group. The ethnicity is identified with an **ethnonym** (see below).

Disadvantaged Background – refers to a citizen, national, or a lawful permanent resident of the United States, the Commonwealths of Puerto Rico or the Marianas Islands, the U.S. Virgin Islands, Guam, American Samoa, the Trust Territory of the Pacific Islands, the Republic of Palau, the Republic of the Marshall Islands, or the Federated State of Micronesia who is:

HRSA defines a "disadvantaged" individual as someone who (a) comes from an environment that has inhibited the individual from obtaining the knowledge, skill, and abilities required to enroll in and graduate from a school (environmentally disadvantaged); or (b) comes from a family with an annual income below a level which is based on low-income thresholds according to family size published by the U.S. Bureau of the Census, adjusted annually for changes in the Consumer Price Index, and adjusted by the Secretary of HHS for adaptation to this program (economically disadvantaged).[27]

Economically Disadvantaged – an individual from a family with an annual income below a level based on low-income thresholds, according to family size established by the U.S. Census Bureau, adjusted annually for changes in the Consumer Price Index, and adjusted by the Secretary of the U.S. Department of Health and Human Services, for use in all health professions programs. A family is a group of two or more individuals. The Secretary updates these income levels in the Federal Register annually AND/OR

Educationally Disadvantaged – an individual who comes from a social, cultural, or educational environment that has demonstrably and directly inhibited the individual from obtaining the knowledge, skills, and abilities necessary to develop and participate in a health professions education or training program.

Environmentally Disadvantaged – an individual's environment inhibited him/her from obtaining the knowledge, skills, and abilities required to enroll in and graduate from a health professions school

Educational attainment – the highest level of education completed by an individual or group

Ethnicity – the ethnic ancestry or origin of an individual or group of individuals. For the purposes of performance reporting, the Office of Management and Budget (OMB) requires you classify ethnicity as "Hispanic or Latino Origin" and "Non-Hispanic or Latino Origin." Individuals identifying as "Hispanic or Latino" are of Cuban, Mexican, Puerto Rican, South or Central American, or other Spanish culture or origin regardless of race.

Ethnonym (from the Greek: éthnos, "nation" and ónoma, "name") – a name applied to a given ethnic group.

Health Disparity Population (HDP) – a population that has a significant disparity in the overall rate of disease incidence, prevalence, morbidity, mortality, or survival rates in the population, as compared to the health status of the general population. It further includes populations for which there is a significant disparity in the quality, outcomes, cost, use of, access to, or satisfaction with health care services, as compared to the general population.

Health inequality- According to the WHO, health inequalities can be defined as differences in health status or in the distribution of health determinants between different population groups. Inequalities can be due to <u>unavoidable</u> factors, such as genetics, and thus be difficult or impossible for the affected individual to change.

Health inequity – Avoidable inequalities in health between groups of people within countries and between countries. These inequities arise from social and economic conditions poor governance, corruption or discrimination. Their effects on people's lives determine their risk of illness and the actions taken to prevent them becoming ill or treat illness when it occurs (World Health Organization).

The difference between the terms inequity and inequality can be difficult to understand. In general, inequality refers primarily to the condition of being unequal, and it can be expressed in numbers. Inequity can be considered as a synonym of injustice and unfairness, so it usually relates to more qualitative matters.

Health Professional Shortage Area (HPSA) – a federal designation used to identify areas, populations, and facilities which have a shortage of either primary care, dental, and/or mental health providers as measured by the ratio of available discipline-specific providers to: the population of the area, a specific population group; or the number of those served by the facility. For primary medical care, the population to provider ratio must be at least 3,500 to 1 (3,000 to 1 if there are unusually high needs in the community) to be considered as having a shortage of providers.

The Medical Admission Test (MCAT) – evaluates most of the courses required for entry to a medical school (physics, organic chemistry, general chemistry, biology, biochemistry, psychology, and sociology along with a section of critical analysis and verbal reasoning.

Medically Underserved Area (MUA) – counties, a group of counties or civil divisions, or a group of urban census tracts in which residents have a shortage of personal health services.

The Medically Underserved Area designation is based on an Index of Medical Underservice, which is derived from an area's ratio of primary medical care physicians per 1,000 population, infant mortality rate, percentage of the population with incomes below the poverty level, and percentage of the population age 65 or over.

Medically Underserved Community (MUC) – a geographic location or population of individuals eligible for designation by the federal government as a Health Professional Shortage Area, Medically Underserved Area, Medically Underserved Population, or Governor's Certified Shortage Area for Rural Health Clinic purposes. As an umbrella term, MUC also includes populations such as homeless individuals, migrant or seasonal workers, and residents of public housing.

Medically Underserved Populations (MUPs) – federally-designated population groups having a shortage of personal health services, often defined as groups who face economic, cultural, or linguistic barriers to health care, and limited access to services. The Index of Medical Underservice designates MUPs.

National Assessment of Educational Progress (NAEP) – measures students' knowledge of three content areas: physical science, life science, and earth and space sciences at grades 4, 8, and 12 in both public and private schools nationwide. NAEP science scores range from 0 to 300 for all three grades.

Promotores - A promotor/promotora is a Hispanic/Latino community member who is not a professional health care worker, but receives specialized training to provide basic health education in the community.

SAT – Introduced in 1926, the "Scholastic Assessment Test" which has been renamed a few times, is the most commonly test taken by high school juniors and seniors before they apply for college admissions. The test assesses reading, writing, and math and may include an optional essay, depending on the institution. The overall scoring scale ranges from 400 to 1600.

Social Determinants of Health – the circumstances in which people are born, grow up, live, work, and age, as well as the systems put in place to deal with illness.

Status completion rate – The NCEs defines it as "the percentage of 18- to 24-year-old young adults in the United States who hold a high school diploma or an alternative credential." "Unlike high school graduation rates, which measure the percentage of students who graduate during a specific school year, status completion rates include all individuals in a specified age range who hold a high school diploma or alternative credential, regardless of when it was attained."

Underrepresented Minority (URM) – an individual from a racial and/or ethnic group considered inadequately represented in a specific profession relative to the representation of that racial and/or ethnic group in the general population. Note: For the purposes of the health professions, we consider individuals from the following racial and ethnic backgrounds underrepresented: American Indian or Alaska Native, Black or African American, Native Hawaiian or Other Pacific Islander, Hispanic (all races). HRSA defines an underrepresented minority as "racial and ethnic populations that are underrepresented in the health professions relative to the number of individuals who are members of the population involved. This definition would include Black or African American, Hispanic or Latino, American Indian or Alaskan Native.

The Index of Medical Underservice designates MUAs as a subset of a Medically Underserved Community. Visit their Medically Underserved Areas and Populations section for more information.

Underrepresented in Medicine – Since 2004, the AAMC has referred to physicians from some racial and ethnic minority groups as being underrepresented in medicine (URM).

Vulnerable Populations – groups of individuals at higher risk for health disparities by virtue of their race or ethnicity, socio-economic status, geography, gender, age, disability status, or other risk factors associated with sex and gender.

TABLE OF FIGURES

Figure 25. percentage of bachelor's degrees conferred in science, technology, engineering, and mathematics (STEM) fields by race and ethnicity, 2016-2017

Figure 26. Hispanic Medical School Applicants by country of origin

Figure 27. U.S. Young Adult Population Versus Medical School Matriculants, By Race And Ethnicity, 2017

Figure 28. Total graduates in U.S. Medical schools by race and ethnicity 2017-2018. The graph does not include all races for simplicity

Figure 29. Residency Applicants from U.S. MD-Granting Medical Schools to ACGME-Accredited Programs by selected Specialty and Race/Ethnicity. The graph shows% of total applicants per specialty The graph does not include all races for simplicity. Created using data from the AAMC

Figure 30. Residency applicants from U.S. MD-granting medical schools by specialty and race/ethnicity 2018-2019

Figure 31. Distribution of Physicians by Race/Ethnicity relative to the working age population (source: HRSA ACS PUMS 2011-2015)

Figure 32. Healthcare Worker drivers for Supply and Demand. Modified from [124] [125] [126]. One of the most important drivers of health workforce supply is the number of medical school graduates.

Box 2. Variables commonly used to define physician shortages

Figure 33. Physicians practicing in underserved areas, by state. (More than half (54.6%) of the individuals who completed their residency training from 2009 through 2018 are practicing in the state where they did their residency training.)

Figure 34. Percent of need met health professional shortage areas, 2019

Figure 35. The educational journey, from elementary school to residency

Figure 36. Risk factors for low educational attainment

Figure 51.Adult Healthcare Literacy by race and ethnicity. Source: US Dept. of Education 2003 [270]

Figure 52. Average health literacy scores of adults, by race/ethnicity: 2003

Figure 53. Teen births by race and ethnicity in the U.S.

Figure 54. A three-step plan towards medical school

REFERENCES

1. Scioscia, *A. Critical Connection*. Phoenix New Times, 2000. Available from: http://www.phoenixnewtimes.com/2000-06-29/news/critical-connection/.

2. Harsham, P., *A misinterpreted word worth 71 million*. J Med Econ, 1984. **61**(12): p. 289-292.

3. Chen, A.H., M.K. Youdelman, and J. Brooks, *The legal framework for language access in healthcare settings: Title VI and beyond*. Journal of general internal medicine, 2007. **22 Suppl 2**(Suppl 2): p. 362-367. Available from: https://www.ncbi.nlm.nih.gov/pmc/articles/PMC2150609/.

4. Quan, K. and J. Lynch, *The High Costs of language barriers in medical malpractice*, S. Lichtman and M. Youdelman, Editors. 2010, University of California, Berkeley.

5. Van Kempen, *A., Legal risks of ineffective communication*. Virtual Mentor, 2007. **9**(8): p. 555-8. Available from: https://www.ncbi.nlm.nih.gov/pubmed/23218150.

6. Passel, J., C. D'Vera, and M. Lopez, *Hispanics Account for More than Half of Nation's Growth in Past Decade*. Journal, 2011. Available from: https://www.pewresearch.org/hispanic/2011/03/24/hispanics-account-for-more-than-half-of-nations-growth-in-past-decade/.

7. Wagner, *A., The Americans Our Government Won't Count*. The New York Times, 2018(March 30). Available from: https://www.nytimes.com/2018/03/30/opinion/sunday/united-states-census.html.

8. Wang, H. *2020 Census Could Lead To Worst Undercount Of Black, Latinx People In 30 Years*. NPR News, 2019. Available from: https://www.npr.org/2019/06/04/728034176/2020-census-could-lead-to-worst-undercount-of-black-latinx-people-in-30-years.

9. Kissam, E., *Differential undercount of Mexican immigrant families in the U.S. census*. Statistical Journal of the International Association of Official Statistics, 2017.

10. Elliott, D., et al., 2020 Census. *Who's at risk of being miscounted?* Urban Insitute, 2019. Available from: http://apps.urban.org/features/2020-census/.

11. Oxford University Press, *Oxford English Dictionary, in Oxford English Dictionary*. Oxford University Press. Available from: https://www.oed.com/.

12. Merriam-Webster. *'Latinx' and the gender inclusivity*. 2018; Available from: https://www.merriam-webster.com/words-at-play/word-history-latinx.

13. Merriam Webster Dictionary. *Merriam Webster Dictionary*. September 12, 2019]; Available from: https://www.merriam-webster.com/dictionary/Hispanic.

14. Learner's Dictionary, Learner's Dictionary. Available from: http://www.learners-dictionary.com/definition/Hispanic.

15. Federal Interagency Committee on Education, *Report of the Ad Hoc Committee on Racial and Ethnic Definitions of the /federal Interagency Committee on Education*. Journal, 1975. Available from: https://files.eric.ed.gov/fulltext/ED121636.pdf.

16. Mora, G.C., *Making Hispanics : how activists, bureaucrats, and media constructed a new American*. 2014, Chicago The University of Chicago Press. Available from: https://www.press.uchicago.edu/ucp/books/book/chicago/M/bo15345128.html.

17. Author The roots of "*Hispanic*". Periodical The roots of "Hispanic", 2003. Available from: https://www.washingtonpost.com/archive/politics/2003/10/15/the-roots-of-hispanic/3d914863-95bc-40f3-9950-ce0c25939046/.

18. National Public Radio, *Who Put The 'Hispanic' In Hispanic Heritage Month?, in Code Switch*. 2017: npr.prg. Available from: https://www.npr.org/sections/codeswitch/2017/09/23/552036578/who-put-the-hispanic-in-hispanic-heritage-month.

19. Carter, C., *Changing Views of Identity in the Face of Globalization Among Hispanic Communities in Diaspora* 2012, Illinois State University.

20. Lopez, M. *Hispanic Identity*. 2013. Available from: https://www.pewresearch.org/hispanic/2013/10/22/3-hispanic-identity/.

21. Waldinger, R. *Transnationalism. Between Here and There: How attached are Latino immigrants to their native country?* Pew Research Center 2007 October 25, 2007; Available from: https://www.pewresearch.org/hispanic/2007/10/25/vi-transnationalism/.

22. O'Hare, W., *Differential Undercounts in the U.S. Census SpringerBriefs in Population Studies*. 2019.

23. Pew Research Center, *What Census Calls Us: A Historical Timeline*. Available from: https://www.pewsocialtrends.org/interactives/multiracial-timeline/.

24. Office of Management and Budget, *Revisions to the Standards for the Classification of Federal Data on Race and Ethnicity*. Federal Register, 1997. 62(210). Available from: https://www.govinfo.gov/content/pkg/FR-1997-10-30/pdf/97-28653.pdf.

25. Pew Research Center. *From Ireland to Germany to Italy to Mexico: How America's Source of Immigrants Has Changed in the States*, 1850 – 2013. 2015; Available from: https://www.pewresearch.org/hispanic/2015/09/28/from-ireland-to-germany-to-italy-to-mexico-how-americas-source-of-immigrants-has-changed-in-the-states-1850-to-2013/.

26. Flores, A., M. Lopez, and J. Krogstad U.S. *Hispanic population reached new high in 2018, but growth has slowed*. FactTank, 2019. Available from: https://www.pewresearch.org/fact-tank/2019/07/08/u-s-hispanic-population-reached-new-high-in-2018-but-growth-has-slowed/.

27. Affirmative Action Program. Report to Congress, *PUBLIC LAW 94-311—JUNE 16, 1976. 1976*. Available from: https://uscode.house.gov/statutes/pl/94/311.pdf.

28. Humes, K.R., N. Jones, and R. Ramirez, *Overview of Race and Hispanic Origin: 2010* U.S. Census Bureau, 2010 Census Brief, 2011. Available from: www.census.gov/prod/cen2010/briefs/c2010br-02.pdf.

29. U.S. Census Bureau. *U.S. Census Bureau, 2013-2017 American Community Survey 5-Year Estimates*. 2017; Available from: https://factfinder.census.gov/faces/tableservices/jsf/pages/productview.xhtml?pid=ACS_17_5YR_DP05&src=pt.

30. Alberti, N., 2005 National Census Test: *Analysis of the Race and Ethnicity Questions*. Census Test Evaluations Memorandum Series. US Census Bureau, 2006.

31. Ríos, M., F. Romero, and R. Ramirez, *Race Reporting Among Hispanics: 2010*. U.S. Census Bureau Working Paper Series 2014(102). Available from: www.census.gov/population/www/documentation/twps0102/twps0102.pdf.

32. Schuster, L., *Race and ethnicity, as measured by the Census*. 2019. Available from: https://www.bostonindicators.org/article-pages/2019/april/race-and-ethnicity-as-measured-by-the-census.

33. Edozie, R., et al., *Changing Faces of Greater Boston*. 2019.

34. Alba, R., *The Likely Persistence of a White Majority. How Census Bureau statistics have misled thinking about the American future.* . The American Prospect 2016. Available from: https://prospect.org/article/likely-persistence-white-majority-0.

35. Compton, E., et al., *2010 Census Race and Hispanic Origin Alternative Questionnaire Experiment*. Journal, 2012. Available from: https://www.census.gov/2010census/pdf/2010_Census_Race_HO_AQE.pdf.

36. Mathews, K., et al., *2015 National Content Test. Race and Ethnicity Analysis Report*. Journal, 2017. Available from: https://www.census.gov/programs-surveys/decennial-census/2020-census/planning-management/final-analysis/2015nct-race-ethnicity-analysis.html.

37. U.S. Census Bureau, *2020 CENSUS PROGRAM MEMORANDUM SERIES*: 2018.06. 2018. Available from: https://www2.census.gov/programs-surveys/

decennial/2020/program-management/memo-series/2020-memo-2018_06.pdf.

38. Baum, M., et al., *Estimating the Effect of Asking About Citizenship on the U.S. Census*. The Shorenstein Center on Media, Politics and Public Policy, 2019.

39. Mellnik, T. and K. Rabinowitz, *Where a citizenship question could cause the census to miss millions of Hispanics. And why that's a big deal*. The Washington Post, 2019(June 27). Available from: https://www.washingtonpost.com/politics/2019/06/06/where-citizenship-question-could-cause-census-miss-millions-hispanics-why-thats-big-deal/?noredirect=on&utm_term=.e990459d426c.

40. Cohn, D. It's official: *Minority babies are the majority among the nation's infants, but only just*. 2016. Available from: https://www.pewresearch.org/fact-tank/2016/06/23/its-official-minority-babies-are-the-majority-among-the-nations-infants-but-only-just/.

41. Lopez, M., A. Gonzales-Barrera, and G. Lopez, *Hispanic Identity Fades Accross generations as immigrant connections fall away,* P.R. Center, Editor. 2017. Available from: https://www.pewresearch.org/hispanic/2017/12/20/hispanic-identity-fades-across-generations-as-immigrant-connections-fall-away/.

42. 42.   Lewontin, R., *The Apportionment of Human Diversity*. Evolutionary Biology. Dobzhansky T., Hecht M.K., Steere W.C. (eds), 1972: p. 381.

43. Barbujani, G., et al., *An apportionment of human DNA diversity*. Proc Natl Acad Sci U S A, 1997. **94**(9): p. 4516-9. Available from: https://www.ncbi.nlm.nih.gov/pubmed/9114021.

44. Marks, J., *The Facts about Human Variation*. Human Evolutionary Biology, ed. M.P. Muehlenbein. 2010: Cambridge University Press.

45. Hubbard, R., *Race & Genes*. Journal, 2006. Available from: http://raceandgenomics.ssrc.org/Hubbard/.

46. Hammonds, E., *Straw Men and Their Followers: The return of biological race*. Journal, 2006. Available from: http://raceandgenomics.ssrc.org/Hammonds/.

47. American Anthropological Association *American Anthropological Association Statement on "Race"*. 1998. Available from: https://www.americananthro.org/ConnectWithAAA/Content.aspx?ItemNumber=2583.

48. Graves, J., *"What We Know and What We Don't Know: Human Genetic Variation and the Social Construction of Race"*. Journal, 2006. Available from: "What We Know and What We Don't Know: Human Genetic Variation and the Social Construction of Race".

49. Duster, T., *Race Identity, in International Encyclopedia of the Social & Behavioral Sciences*, N.J. Smelser and P.B. Baltes, Editors. 2001, Pergamon: Oxford. p. 12703-12706. Available from: http://www.sciencedirect.com/science/article/pii/B0080430767019513.

50. Broman, C.L., *Race Identity, in International Encyclopedia of the Social & Behavioral Sciences (Second Edition)*, J.D. Wright, Editor. 2015, Elsevier: Oxford. p. 833-836. Available from: http://www.sciencedirect.com/science/article/pii/B9780080970868321201.

51. Fukuyama, F., *Identity : the demand for dignity and the politics of resentment*. First edition. ed. 2018, New York: Farrar, Straus and Giroux. xvii, 218 pages.

52. Croll, P.R. and J. Gerteis, *Race as an Open Field: Exploring Identity beyond Fixed Choices*. Sociology of Race and Ethnicity, 2017. 5(1): p. 55-69. Available from: https://doi.org/10.1177/2332649217748425.

53. Parker, K., et al., *Multiracial in America*. 2015. Available from: https://www.pewresearch.org/hispanic/dataset/2014-national-survey-of-latinos/.

54. Pew Research Center. *2015 National Survey of Latinos*. 2015; Available from: https://www.pewresearch.org/hispanic/dataset/2015-national-survey-of-latinos/.

55. Lopez, M., A. Gonzalez-Barrera, and G. López, *"Hispanic Identity Fades Across Generations as Immigrant Connections Fall Away"*. Pew Research Center, 2017.

56. Pew Research Center, *Second-Generation Americans. A portrait of the adult children of immigrants*. Journal, 2013.

57. Parker, K., et al. *Chapter 7: The Many Dimensions of Hispanic Racial Identity*. 2015. Available from: https://www.pewsocialtrends.org/2015/06/11/chapter-7-the-many-dimensions-of-hispanic-racial-identity/.

58. Macintosh, T., et al., *Socially-assigned race, healthcare discrimination and preventive healthcare services*. PLoS One, 2013. 8(5): p. e64522. Available from: https://www.ncbi.nlm.nih.gov/pubmed/23704992.

59. Vargas, E.D., G.R. Sanchez, and B.L. Kinlock, *The Enhanced Self-Reported Health Outcome Observed in Hispanics/Latinos Who are Socially-Assigned as White is Dependent on Nativity*. J Immigr Minor Health, 2015. 17(6): p. 1803-10. Available from: https://www.ncbi.nlm.nih.gov/pubmed/25410381.

60. Krogstad, J., L. M, and M. Rohal, *English Proficiency on the rise among Latinos. U.S. born driving language changes*. Pew Research Center, 2015(May).

61. Lopez, M. *Is speaking Spanish necessary to be Hispanic? Most Hispanics say no*. Factank 2015; Available from: https://www.pewresearch.org/facttank/2016/02/19/is-speaking-spanish-necessary-to-be-hispanic-most-hispanics-say-no/.

62. Alonso, J., J. Durand, and R. Gutierrez, *THE FUTURE OF SPANISH IN THE UNITED STATES: THE LANGUAGE OF HISPANIC MIGRANT COMMUNITIES*. First Edition ed. 2014: Editorial Ariel.

63. National Center for Education Statistics. *Interpreting NAEP Reading Results*. Available from: https://nces.ed.gov/rationsreportcard/reading/interpret_results.aspx.

64. Ho, P. and G. Kao, *Educational Achievement and Attainment Differences Among Minorities and Immigrants. , in Handbook of the Sociology of Education in the 21st Century. Handbooks of Sociology and Social Research.* , B. Schneider, Editor. 2018, Springer.

65. Jaschik, S., SAT Scores *Are Up, Especially for Asians, in Inside Higher Ed. 2018*. Available from: https://www.insidehighered.com/admissions/article/2018/10/29/sat-scores-are-gaps-remain-significant-among-racial-and-ethnic-groups.

66. California Assessment of Student Performance and Progress. *California Science Test (CAST)*. 2020; Available from: https://caaspp-elpac.cde.ca.gov/caaspp/DashViewReportCAST?ps=true&lstTestYear=2019&lstTestType=X-&lstGroup=1&lstSubGroup=1&lstSchoolType=A&lstGrade=13&lstCounty=00&lstDistrict=00000&lstSchool=0000000.

67. Rattani, S., SAT: *Does racial bias exist?* Creative Education, 2016. 7: p. 2151-2162.

68. Aronson, J. and M. Inzlicht, *The ups and downs of attributional ambiguity: stereotype vulnerability and the academic self-knowledge of African American college students.* Psychol Sci, 2004. 15(12): p. 829-36. Available from: https://www.ncbi.nlm.nih.gov/pubmed/15563328.

69. Steele, C.M. and J.A. Aronson, *Stereotype threat does not live by Steele and Aronson (1995) alone.* Am Psychol, 2004. 59(1): p. 47-8; discussion 48-9. Available from: https://www.ncbi.nlm.nih.gov/pubmed/14736323.

70. Steele, C.M. and J. Aronson, *Stereotype threat and the intellectual test performance of African Americans.* J Pers Soc Psychol, 1995. 69(5): p. 797-811. Available from: https://www.ncbi.nlm.nih.gov/pubmed/7473032.

71. Koenig, J.A., S.G. Sireci, and A. Wiley, *Evaluating the predictive validity of MCAT scores across diverse applicant groups.* Acad Med, 1998. 73(10): p. 1095-106. Available from: https://www.ncbi.nlm.nih.gov/pubmed/9795629.

72. Lucey, C.R. and A. Saguil, *The Consequences of Structural Racism on MCAT Scores and Medical School Admissions*: The Past Is Prologue. Acad Med, 2020. 95(3): p. 351-356. Available from: https://www.ncbi.nlm.nih.gov/pubmed/31425184.

73. Jencks, C., *The Black-White Test score gap,* ed. C. Jencks. 1998: RR Donnelly & sons.

74. Author *SAT to Give Students 'Adversity Score' to Capture Social and Economic Background*. Periodical SAT to Give Students 'Adversity Score' to Capture Social and Economic Background, 2019. Available from: https://www.wsj.com/arti-

cles/sat-to-give-students-adversity-score-to-capture-social-and-economic-back-ground-11557999000.

75. Author *SAT's New 'Adversity Score' Will Take Students' Hardships Into Account*. Periodical SAT's New 'Adversity Score' Will Take Students' Hardships Into Account, 2019. Available from: https://nyti.ms/2Q9zPXy.

76. Author *SAT 'Adversity Score' Is Abandoned in Wake of Criticism*. Periodical SAT 'Adversity Score' Is Abandoned in Wake of Criticism, 2019. Available from: https://nyti.ms/2ZrVP6V.

77. Graf, N. *Most Americans say colleges should not consider race or ethnicity in admissions In: Race in America 2019*. FactTank, 2019. Available from: https://www.pewresearch.org/fact-tank/2019/02/25/most-americans-say-colleges-should-not-consider-race-or-ethnicity-in-admissions/.

78. Julian, E.R., *Validity of the Medical College Admission Test for predicting medical school performance*. Acad Med, 2005. **80**(10): p. 910-7. Available from: https://www.ncbi.nlm.nih.gov/pubmed/16186610.

79. Sedlacek, W.E. and D.O. Prieto, *Predicting minority students' success in medical school*. Acad Med, 1990. 65(3): p. 161-6. Available from: https://www.ncbi.nlm.nih.gov/pubmed/2407258.

80. Patterson, F., et al., *How effective are selection methods in medical education? A systematic review*. Med Educ, 2016. 50(1): p. 36-60. Available from: https://www.ncbi.nlm.nih.gov/pubmed/26695465.

81. Patterson, F., L. Zibarras, and V. Ashworth, *Situational judgement tests in medical education and training*: Research, theory and practice: AMEE Guide No. 100. Med Teach, 2016. 38(1): p. 3-17. Available from: https://www.ncbi.nlm.nih.gov/pubmed/26313700.

82. Puma, M.J., et al., *Prospects: Final report on student outcomes*. Journal, 1997. Available from: https://files.eric.ed.gov/fulltext/ED413411.pdf.

83. Collier, C., *Seven Steps to Separating Difference From Disability*. 2011: Corwin Press.

84. Case, R. and S. Taylor, *Language difference or learning disability? Answers from a linguistic perspective*. The Clearing House, 2005. **78**(3): p. 127-131.

85. Barr, R., R. Dreeben, and N. Wiratchai, *How schools work*. 1983, Chicago: University of Chicago Press. xiii, 191 p.; Available from: https://www.press. uchicago.edu/ucp/books/book/chicago/H/bo22957290.html.

86. Taylor, P., et al. *America's Changing workforce. Attitudes Towards Work. 2009*. Available from: https://www.pewsocialtrends.org/2009/09/03/iii-attitudes-to-ward-work/.

87. de Brey, C., et al., *Status and Trends in the Education of Racial and Ethnic Groups 2018 (NCES 2019-038)*. Journal, 2019. Available from: https://nces. ed.gov/pubsearch/.

88. Hussar, W.J. and T.M. Bailey, *Projections of Education Statistics to 2027 (NCES 2019-001)*. Journal, 2019. Available from: https://nces.ed.gov/pubs2019/2019001.pdf.

89. Rumberger, R.W., *Dropping out : why students drop out of high school and what can be done about it*. 2011, Cambridge, Mass.: Harvard University Press. xii, 380 p.

90. Steinberg, L., P. Blinde, and K. Chan, *Dropping out among language minority youth*. Review of Educational Research, 1984. **54**: p. 113-132.

91. Gurin, P., *Expert Report of Patricia Gurin*. 5 Mich. J. Race & L. , 1999. 5(363).

92. Alexander, C., E. Chen, and K. Grumbach, *How leaky is the health career pipeline? Minority student achievement in college gateway courses*. Acad Med, 2009. 84(6): p. 797-802. Available from: https://www.ncbi.nlm.nih.gov/pubmed/19474563.

93. Khan, N.R., C.M. Taylor, 2nd, and K.L. Rialon, *Resident Perspectives on the Current State of Diversity in Graduate Medical Education*. J Grad Med Educ,

2019. 11(2): p. 241-243. Available from: https://www.ncbi.nlm.nih.gov/pubmed/31024664.

94. Pololi, L., L.A. Cooper, and P. Carr, *Race, disadvantage and faculty experiences in academic medicine*. J Gen Intern Med, 2010. 25(12): p. 1363-9. Available from: https://www.ncbi.nlm.nih.gov/pubmed/20697960.

95. Yu, P.T., et al., *Minorities struggle to advance in academic medicine: A 12-y review of diversity at the highest levels of America's teaching institutions*. J Surg Res, 2013. 182(2): p. 212-8. Available from: https://www.ncbi.nlm.nih.gov/pubmed/23582226.

96. Adanga, E., et al., *An environmental scan of faculty diversity programs at U.S. medical schools*. Acad Med, 2012. 87(11): p. 1540-7. Available from: https://www.ncbi.nlm.nih.gov/pubmed/23018325.

97. Lin, S.Y., et al., *Faculty diversity and inclusion program outcomes at an academic otolaryngology department*. Laryngoscope, 2016. 126(2): p. 352-6. Available from: https://www.ncbi.nlm.nih.gov/pubmed/26153871.

98. Price, E.G., et al., *The role of cultural diversity climate in recruitment, promotion, and retention of faculty in academic medicine*. J Gen Intern Med, 2005. **20**(7): p. 565-71. Available from: https://www.ncbi.nlm.nih.gov/pubmed/16050848.

99. Guevara, J.P., et al., *The Harold Amos Medical Faculty Development Program: Evaluation of a National Program to Promote Faculty Diversity and Health Equity*. Health Equity, 2018. **2**(1): p. 7-14. Available from: https://www.ncbi.nlm.nih.gov/pubmed/30283846.

100. Nivet, M.A., *Minorities in academic medicine: review of the literature*. J Vasc Surg, 2010. **51**(4 Suppl): p. 53S-58S. Available from: https://www.ncbi.nlm.nih.gov/pubmed/20036099.

101. Page, K.R., L. Castillo-Page, and S.M. Wright, *Faculty diversity programs in U.S. medical schools and characteristics associated with higher faculty diversity*. Acad Med, 2011. **86**(10): p. 1221-8. Available from: https://www.ncbi.nlm.nih.gov/pubmed/21869663.

102. Rice, T.K., et al., *Enhancing the Careers of Under-Represented Junior Faculty in Biomedical Research: The Summer Institute Program to Increase Diversity (SIPID)*. J Natl Med Assoc, 2014. **106**(1): p. 50-57. Available from: https://www.ncbi.nlm.nih.gov/pubmed/25684827.

103. Efstathiou, J.A., et al., *Long-term impact of a faculty mentoring program in academic medicine*. PLoS One, 2018. **13**(11): p. e0207634. Available from: https://www.ncbi.nlm.nih.gov/pubmed/30496199.

104. Choi, A.M.K., et al., *Developing a Culture of Mentorship to Strengthen Academic Medical Centers*. Acad Med, 2019. **94**(5): p. 630-633. Available from: https://www.ncbi.nlm.nih.gov/pubmed/31026234.

105. Pace, B.S., et al., *Enhancing diversity in the hematology biomedical research workforce: A mentoring program to improve the odds of career success for early stage investigators*. Am J Hematol, 2017. **92**(12): p. 1275-1279. Available from: https://www.ncbi.nlm.nih.gov/pubmed/28857249.

106. Pololi, L. and S. Knight, *Mentoring faculty in academic medicine. A new paradigm?* J Gen Intern Med, 2005. **20**(9): p. 866-70. Available from: https://www.ncbi.nlm.nih.gov/pubmed/16117759.

107. Osman, N.Y. and B. Gottlieb, *Mentoring Across Differences*. MedEdPORTAL, 2018. **14**: p. 10743. Available from: https://www.ncbi.nlm.nih.gov/pubmed/30800943.

108. Ortega, G., et al., *Preparing for an Academic Career: The Significance of Mentoring*. MedEdPORTAL, 2018. 14: p. 10690. Available from: https://www.ncbi.nlm.nih.gov/pubmed/30800890.

109. Organization, W.H., *Global Reference List of 100 Core Health Indicators*. Journal, 2018. Available from: https://apps.who.int/iris/bitstream/handle/10665/259951/WHO-HIS-IER-GPM-2018.1-eng.pdf;jsessionid=7DC11EA8D-D6C5C40010E34D7571A45AA?sequence=1.

110. Sanchez, G., et al., *Latino Physicians in the United States, 1980-2010: A Thirty-Year Overview From the Censuses*. Acad Med., 2015. **90**: p. 906-912.

111. Salsberg, E., *Annual State of the Physician Workforce address*. AAMC. 2009. Journal, 2013. Available from: https://www.aamc.org/download/82844/data/annualaddress09.pdf.

112. Iglehart, J.K., *The residency mismatch*. N Engl J Med, 2013. **369**(4): p. 297-9. Available from: https://www.ncbi.nlm.nih.gov/pubmed/23782122.

113. Colleges, A.o.A.M., *The Complexities of Physician Supply and Demand. Projections from 2017 to 2032*. Journal, 2019. Available from: https://www.aamc.org/system/files/c/2/31-2019_update_-_the_complexities_of_physician_supply_and_demand_-_projections_from_2017-2032.pdf.

114. Colleges, A.o.A.M., *Myths and Facts: The Physician Shortage. Journal, 2019*. Available from: https://www.aamc.org/system/files/2019-09/myths-facts-physician-shortage-2019-Apr.pdf.

115. Institute of Medicine, *Graduate Medical Education That Meets the Nation's Health Needs*. Graduate Medical Education That Meets the Nation's Health Needs, ed. J. Eden, D. Berwick, and G. Wilensky. 2014, Washington (DC): Institute of Medicine. Committee on the Governance and Financing of Graduate Medical Education. Available from: https://www.ncbi.nlm.nih.gov/pubmed/25340242.

116. Ryan, C. Doc *Shortage or Maldistribution?* AAF Weekly Checkup, 2014. Available from: http://americanactionforum.aaf.rededge.com/uploads/files/serialized_products/Weekly_Checkup_20140814.pdf.

117. Xierali, I.M. and M.A. Nivet, *The Racial and Ethnic Composition and Distribution of Primary Care Physicians*. J Health Care Poor Underserved, 2018. 29(1): p. 556-570. Available from: https://www.ncbi.nlm.nih.gov/pubmed/29503317.

118. Komaromy, M., et al., *The role of black and Hispanic physicians in providing health care for underserved populations*. N Engl J Med, 1996. **334**(20): p. 1305-10. Available from: https://www.ncbi.nlm.nih.gov/pubmed/8609949.

119. Martinez, L., et al., *The Current State of the Latino Physician Workforce: A policy series generously supported by California Faces a Severe Shortfall in Latino Resident Physicians*. Journal, 2019.

120. Grumbach, K. and R. Mendoza, *Disparities in human resources: addressing the lack of diversity in the health professions.* Health Aff (Millwood), 2008. **27**(2): p. 413-22. Available from: https://www.ncbi.nlm.nih.gov/pubmed/18332497.

121. Terrell, C. and J. Beaudreau, *3000 by 2000 and beyond: next steps for promoting diversity in the health professions.* J Dent Educ, 2003. **67**(9): p. 1048-52. Available from: https://www.ncbi.nlm.nih.gov/pubmed/14518847.

122. Kelly-Blake, K., et al., *Rationales for expanding minority physician representation in the workforce: a scoping review.* Med Educ, 2018. Available from: https://www.ncbi.nlm.nih.gov/pubmed/29932213.

123. Institute of Medicine, *Unequal Treatment: Confronting Racial and Ethnic Disparities in Health Care (with CD)*, ed. B.D. Smedley, A.Y. Stith, and A.R. Nelson. 2003, Washington, DC: The National Academies Press. 432. Available from: https://www.nap.edu/catalog/12875/unequal-treatment-confronting-racial-and-ethnic-disparities-in-health-care.

124. Sullivan, L.W., *Missing Persons: Minorities in the Health Professions, A Report of the Sullivan Commission on Diversity in the Healthcare Workforce.* Journal, 2004. Available from: http://health-equity.lib.umd.edu/40/.

125. Reede, J., *Letter to the Editor.* JAMA, 2014. **311**(11): p. 1157.

126. Author *UC admits largest and most diverse class ever of Californian freshmen.* Periodical UC admits largest and most diverse class ever of Californian freshmen, 2019. Available from: https://www.latimes.com/california/story/2019-07-22/uc-diverse-diversity-class-student-admissions.

127. Grumbach, K. and E. Chen, *Effectiveness of University of California postbaccalaureate premedical programs in increasing medical school matriculation for minority and disadvantaged students.* JAMA, 2006. **296**(9): p. 1079-85. Available from: https://www.ncbi.nlm.nih.gov/pubmed/16954487.

128. Harvard College. *Admissions Statistics.* 2019; Available from: https://college.harvard.edu/admissions/admissions-statistics.

129. Winkleby, M.A., et al., *Increasing Diversity in Science and Health Professions: A 21-Year Longitudinal Study Documenting College and Career Success*. Journal of Science Education and Technology. 2009. **18**(6): p. 535-545. Available from: https://doi.org/10.1007/s10956-009-9168-0.

130. Cantor, J.C., L. Bergeisen, and L.C. Baker, *Effect of an intensive educational program for minority college students and recent graduates on the probability of acceptance to medical school*. JAMA, 1998. **280**(9): p. 772-6. Available from: https://www.ncbi.nlm.nih.gov/pubmed/9729987.

131. Smith, S.G., et al., *Pipeline programs in the health professions, part 2: the impact of recent legal challenges to affirmative action*. J Natl Med Assoc, 2009. **101**(9): p. 852-63. Available from: https://www.ncbi.nlm.nih.gov/pubmed/19806841.

132. Smith, S.G., et al., *Pipeline programs in the health professions, part 1: preserving diversity and reducing health disparities*. J Natl Med Assoc, 2009. **101**(9): p. 836-40, 845-51. Available from: https://www.ncbi.nlm.nih.gov/pubmed/19806840.

133. Butler, P., et al., *The Diverse Surgeons Initiative: An Effective Method for Increasing the number of under-represented minorities in Academic Surgery*. Journal of the American College of Surgeons, 2010. **211**(4): p. 561-565.

134. Jolly, P., C. Erikson, and G. Garrison, *U.S. graduate medical education and physician specialty choice*. Acad Med, 2013. **88**(4): p. 468-74. Available from: https://www.ncbi.nlm.nih.gov/pubmed/23425979.

135. Committee on the Governance and Financing of Graduate Medical Education; Board on Health Care Services; Institute of Medicine, *Background on the Pipeline to the Physician Workforce, in Graduate Medical Education That Meets the Nation's Health Needs*, Eden J, Berwick D, and W. G, Editors. 2014, National Academies Press (US). Available from: https://www.ncbi.nlm.nih.gov/books/NBK248023/.

136. Program, N.R.M., *U.S. Medical Students Learn 2014 National Resident Matching Program® (NRMP®)*. 2014. Available from: http://www.nrmp.org/wp-content/

uploads/2014/03/2014-National-Resident-Matching-Program-NRMP-Main-Res-idency-Match-Results-Press-Release.pdf.

137. Crosby, F.J., A. Iyer, and S. Sincharoen, *Understanding affirmative action. Annu Rev Psychol*, 2006. 57: p. 585-611. Available from: https://www.ncbi.nlm.nih.gov/pubmed/16318608.

138. Bowen, W. and D. Bok, *The Shape of the River: Long-Term Consequences of Considering Race in College and University Admissions*. 1998: Princeton University Press.

139. Gladwell, M., *Malcolm Gladwell, David and Goliath: Underdogs, Misfits, and the Art of Battling Giants*. 2009: Little Brown and Company.

140. Jack, A.A., *The Privileged Poor: How Elite Colleges Are Failing Disadvantaged Students* 1st Edition ed. 2019: Harvard University Press.

141. Bergmann, B., *In defense of affirmative action*. 1996, New York: Basuc Books.

142. Berry, R., *Affirmative action in higher education: Costs, benefits, and implementation*. Journal of public budgeting, accounting & financial management, 2004. **16**(2): p. 257-276. Available from: https://pdfs.semanticscholar.org/80f7/c0e-886011b37396e136eb61b8d659c1c0fe5.pdf.

143. Magnus, S.A. and S.S. Mick, *Medical schools, affirmative action, and the neglected role of social class*. Am J Public Health, 2000. **90**(8): p. 1197-201. Available from: https://www.ncbi.nlm.nih.gov/pubmed/10936995.

144. Lakhan, S.E., *Diversification of U.S. medical schools via affirmative action implementation*. BMC Med Educ, 2003. 3: p. 6. Available from: https://www.ncbi.nlm.nih.gov/pubmed/13678423.

145. Chavez, L. *Affirmative action doctors can kill you. Jewish World Review*, 2001. Available from: http://www.jewishworldreview.com/cols/chavez062101.asp.

146. Carlisle, D.M., J.E. Gardner, and H. Liu, *The entry of underrepresented minority students into US medical schools: an evaluation of recent trends*. Am J Public

Health, 1998. **88**(9): p. 1314-8. Available from: https://www.ncbi.nlm.nih.gov/pubmed/9736869.

147. Chapman, C.H., et al., *Current status of diversity by race, Hispanic ethnicity, and sex in diagnostic radiology*. Radiology, 2014. **270**(1): p. 232-40. Available from: https://www.ncbi.nlm.nih.gov/pubmed/23901125.

148. Chapman, C.H., W.T. Hwang, and C. Deville, *Diversity based on race, ethnicity, and sex, of the US radiation oncology physician workforce*. Int J Radiat Oncol Biol Phys, 2013. **85**(4): p. 912-8. Available from: https://www.ncbi.nlm.nih.gov/pubmed/23122983.

149. Landry, A.M., et al., *Under-represented minorities in emergency medicine*. J Emerg Med, 2013. **45**(1): p. 100-4. Available from: https://www.ncbi.nlm.nih.gov/pubmed/23490110.

150. Day, C.S., D.E. Lage, and C.S. Ahn, *Diversity based on race, ethnicity, and sex between academic orthopaedic surgery and other specialties: a comparative study*. J Bone Joint Surg Am, 2010. **92**(13): p. 2328-35. Available from: https://www.ncbi.nlm.nih.gov/pubmed/20926728.

151. Rayburn, W.F., et al., *Racial and Ethnic Differences Between Obstetrician-Gyne-cologists and Other Adult Medical Specialists*. Obstet Gynecol, 2016. **127**(1): p. 148-52. Available from: https://www.ncbi.nlm.nih.gov/pubmed/26646119.

152. Xierali, I.M., M.A. Nivet, and M.R. Wilson, *Current and Future Status of Diversity in Ophthalmologist Workforce*. JAMA Ophthalmol, 2016. **134**(9): p. 1016-23. Available from: https://www.ncbi.nlm.nih.gov/pubmed/27416525.

153. Health Workforce Research, *Program on Health Workforce Research and Policy. Developing an open-source model for projecting physician shortages in the United States,*. Journal, 2012. Available from: https://www.shepscenter.unc.edu/workforce_product/developing-open-source-model-projecting-physi-cian-shortages-united-states/.

154. Pungello, E., et al., *Early Educational Intervention, Early Cumulative Risk, and the Early Home Environment as Predictors of Young Adult Outcomes Within*

a High-Risk Sample. Child Development, 2010. **81**(1): p. 410. Available from: http://onlinelibrary.wiley.com/doi/10.1111/j.1467-8624.2009.01403.x/full. .

155. Karberg, E., et al., *Family stability and instability among low-income Hispanic mothers with young children*. Journal, 2017. Available from: http://www.hispanicresearchcenter.org/publications/family-stability-and-instability-among-low-income-hispanicmothers-with-young-children/.

156. Wildsmith, E., M. Ramos-Olazagasti, and M. Alvira-Hammond, *The Job Characteristics of Low-Income Hispanic Parents*. Journal, 2018. Available from: https://www.hispanicresearchcenter.org/wp-content/uploads/2019/08/Hispanics-Center-Employment-Profiles-FINAL1.pdf.

157. Gennetian, L., et al., *Income instability in the lives of Hispanic children*. Journal, 2015. Available from: http://www.hispanicresearchcenter.org/publications/income-instability-in-the-lives-of-hispanic-children/.

158. Rojas-Flores, L. *Latino US-Citizen Children of Immigrants: A Generation at High Risk. Summary of Selected Young Scholars Program Research*. 2017.

159. 159. Pew Trusts. 2011; Available from: https://www.pewtrusts.org/en/projects/archived-projects/pre-k-now.

160. Cabrera, N. and A. Hennigar, *The Early Home Environment of Latino Children: A Research Synthesis*. Report 2019-20-45. Journal, 2019. Available from: http://www.hispanicresearchcenter.org/publications/the-earlyhome-environment-of-latino-children-a-research-synthesis.

161. Votruba-Drzal, E., et al., *Center-Based Preschool and School Readiness Skills of Children from Immigrant Families*. Early Education and Development, 2015. **26**(4).

162. Vitaro, F., *Linkages between early childhood, school success, and high school completion. Encyclopedia on Early Childhood Development*, 2014. Available from: http://www.child-encyclopedia.com/sites/default/files/textes-experts/en/839/linkages-between-early-childhood-school-success-and-high-school-completion.pdf.

163. Bakken, L., N. Brown, and B. Downing, *Early Childhood Education: The Long-Term Benefits, Journal of Research in Childhood Education*. 2017. **31**(2): p. 255.

164. Smith, A. *School Completion/Academic Achievement-Outcomes of Early Childhood Education*. 2014. School Success. Available from: http://www.child-encyclopedia.com/sites/default/files/textes-experts/en/839/school-completionacademic-achievement-outcomes-of-ear y-childhood-education.pdf.

165. De Brey, C., et al., *Status and trends in the education of racial and ethnic groups 2018*. 2019, U.S. Department of Education. National Center for Education statistics. Available from: https://nces ed.gov/pubsearch/.

166. Galvez, M., et al., *Associations Between Neighborhood Resources and Physical Activity in Inner-City Minority Children*. Acad. Pediatr., 2013. 13: p. 20-26.

167. Ramirez, A., et al. *The state of Latino early childhood development: A research review*. Salud America, 2017. Available from: https://salud-america.org/wp-content/uploads/2017/11/Early-Child-Dev-Res-Review.pdf.

168. Vikraman, S., C. Fryar, and C. Ogden *Caloric intake from fast food among children and adolescents in the United States*, 2011-2012. NCHS Data Brief, 2012.

169. Liu, G., et al., *The obesity epidemic in children: Latino children are disproportionately affected at younger ages*. Int. J. Pediatr. Adolesc. Med., 2015. 2: p. 12-18.

170. Stephen, C. and R. Monique, *The Influence of Race-Ethnicity and Physical Activity Levels on Elementary School Achievement*. Journal of Educational Research, 2018. **111**(4): p. 473-486.

171. Hanson, M.J., et al., *Neighborhood Community Risk Influences on Preschool Children's Development and School Readiness*. 2011. **24**(1): p. 87-100. Available from: https://journals.lww.com/iycjournal/Fulltext/2011/01000/Neighborhood_Community_Risk_Influences_on.7.aspx.

172. Youngclaus, J. and L. Roskovensky, *An updated look at the economic diversity of U.S. medical students*. Journal, 2018. 18.

173. Musick, K. and A. Meier, *Are both parents always better than one? Parental conflict and young adult well-being*. Soc Sci Res, 2010. 39(5): p. 814-30. Available from: https://www.ncbi.nlm.nih.gov/pubmed/20824195.

174. Murphey, D., L. Guzman, and A. Torres, *America's Hispanic Children: Gaining Ground, Looking Forward. Journal*, 2014. Available from: https://www.childtrends.org/publications/americas-hispanic-children-gaining-ground-looking-forward

175. Banerjee, P.A., *A systematic review of factors linked to poor academic performance of disadvantaged students in science and maths in schools*. Cogent Education, 2016. **3**(1). Available from: http://doi.org/10.1080/2331186X.2016.1178441.

176. Corcoran, L. and S. Grady, **Early Childhood Program Participation, Results from the National Household Education Surveys Program of 2016**. First Look Journal, 2019. Available from: https://nces.ed.gov/pubs2017/2017101REV.pdf.

177. Division, U.S.C.B.D.S.S., *Investigating the 2010 Undercount of Young Children – A Comparison of Demographic, Housing, and Household Characteristics of Children by Age. Journal*, 2017(January, 18 2017). Available from: https://www2.census.gov/programs-surveys/decennial/2020/program-management/final-analysis-reports/2020-2017_02-UndercountofYoungChildrenReport.pdf.

178. Genesee, F., et al., *English Language Learners in U.S. Schools: An overview of research findings*. Journal of Education for Students placed at risk, 2005. 10: p. 363. Available from: https://www.tandfonline.com/doi/abs/10.1207/s15327671espr1004_2.

179. Pryor, J., et al., *T-he American Freshman: Forty year trends, 1966-2006*. Journal, 2007.

180. Grimm, R., E. Solari, and M. Gerber, *A longitudinal investigation of reading development from kindergarten to grade eight in a Spanish-speaking bilingual population*. Read Writ, 2018. 31: p. 559.

181. Gandara, P.C. and F. Contreras, *The Latino education crisis : the consequences of failed social policies. 2009, Cambridge, Mass.: Harvard University Press*.

415 p.; Available from: Table of contents only http://www.loc.gov/catdir/toc/ecip0820/2008024118.html.

182. Burrus, J. and R. Roberts *Dropping Out of High School: Prevalence, Risk Factors, and Remediation Strategies. R&D Connections*, 2012. Available from: https://www.ets.org/Media/Research/pdf/RD_Connections18.pdf.

183. Yu, F. and D. Patterson, *Examining Adolescent Academic Achievement: A Cross-Cultural Review.* The Family Journal, 2010. **18**(3).

184. Faircloth, B. and J. Hamm, *Sense of Belonging Among High School Students Representing four Ethnic Groups.* Journal of Youth and Adolescence, 2005. **34**(4): p. 33-48.

185. Difo, O., *Encouraging Latino Students through Relational Teaching: A Case Study in Lawrence,* Massachusetts. 2015, Concordia University- Portland. Available from: https://pdfs.semanticscholar.org/e98d/194368eaac982bcc26fff-91094d3283281a4.pdf.

186. Belfield, C., H. Levin, and R. Rosen, *The Economic Value of Opportunity Youth. Corporation for National and Community Service and the White House Council for Community Solutions*, 2012. Available from: https://aspencommunityso-lutions.org/wp-content/uploads/2018/07/Economic_Value_of_Opportuni-ty_Youth_Report.pdf.

187. Bridgeland, J., J. Dijulio, and K. Burke, *The Silent Epidemic: Perspectives of High School Dropouts*. Journal, 2006. Available from: https://files.eric.ed.gov/full-text/ED513444.pdf.

188. Choi, A., et al., *Developing a Culture of Mentorship to Strenghten Academic Medical Centers.* Acad Med., 2019. **94**(5): p. 630-633.

189. Johnson, J., B. Williams, and R. Jayadevappa, *Mentoring program for minority faculty at the University of Pennsylvania School of Medicine.* Acad Med., 1999. **74**(4): p. 376-379.

190. Efstathiou, J., et al., *Long-term impact of faculty mentoring program in academ-ic medicine*. PLoS One, 2018. **13**(11): p e0207634.

191. LH, P., et al., *A novel measure of "good" mentoring: testing its reliability and validity in four academic health centers.* J Contin Educ Health Prof, 2016. **36**(4): p. 263-268.

192. Health, N.I.o., *Draft Report of the Advisory Committee to the Director Working Group on Diversity in the Biomedical Research Workforce.* 2012. Available from: https://acd.od.nih.gov/documents/reports/DiversityBiomedicalResearchWorkforceReport.pdf.

193. Jamboor Vishwanatha, C., E. Pfund, and O. Kolawole, *NIH's mentoring makes progress.* Science Magazine, 2016. **354**(6314): p. 840-841.

194. Rice, T., et al., *Mentored Training to increase diversity among faculty in the biomedical sciences: The NHLBI Summer Institute Programs to Increase Diversity (SIPID) and the Programs to Increase Diversity among Individuals Engaged in health-related research (PRIDE).* Ethnicity and Disease, 2017. **27**(3): p. 249-256.

195. Pace, B., et al., *Enhancing diversity in the hematology biomedical research workforce: A mentoring program to improve the odds of career success for early stage investigators.* Am. J. Hematol., 2017. **92**(12): p. 1275-1279.

196. Rice, T., et al., *Enhancing the Careers of Under-represented junior faculty in Biomedical Research: The Summer Institute Program to Increase Diversity* (SIPID). J Natl. Med. Assoc., 2014. **106**(1): p. 50-57.

197. Boyington, J.E., et al., *A Perspective on Promoting Diversity in the Biomedical Research Workforce: The National Heart, Lung, and Blood Institute's PRIDE Program.* Ethn Dis, 2016. **26**(3): p. 379-86. Available from: https://www.ncbi.nlm.nih.gov/pubmed/27440978.

198. Nelson Laird, T.F.J.R.i.H.E., *College Students' Experiences with Diversity and Their Effects on Academic Self-Confidence, Social Agency, and Disposition toward Critical Thinking.* 2005. **46**(4): p. 365-387. Available from: https://doi.org/10.1007/s11162-005-2966-1.

199. Mickelson, R.A. and M. Nkomo, *Integrated Schooling, Life Course Outcomes, and Social Cohesion in Multiethnic Democratic Societies.* 2012.

36(1): p. 197-238. Available from: https://journals.sagepub.com/doi/abs/10.3102/0091732X11422667.

200. Wells, A.S. and R.L. Crain, *Perpetuation Theory and the Long-Term Effects of School Desegregation*. 1994. **64**(4): p. 531-555. Available from: https://journals.sagepub.com/doi/abs/10.3102/00346543064004531.

201. Frankenberg, E., *The Role of Residential Segregation in Contemporary School Segregation*. 2013. **45**(5): p. 548-570. Available from: https://journals.sagepub.com/doi/abs/10.1177/0013124513486288.

202. Fuller, B., et al., *Worsening School Segregation for Latino Children?* 2019. **48**(7): p. 407-420. Available from: https://journals.sagepub.com/doi/abs/10.3102/0013189X19860814.

203. Stewart, P. Scholars *Examine Segregation of Latino K-12 Students*. Diverse Education, 2019. Available from: https://diverseeducation.com/article/156524/.

204. Adelman, C., *Answers in the tool box : academic intensity, attendance patterns, and bachelor's degree attainment*. 1999, Washington, DC (Washington 20208-5531) Jessup, Md.: U.S. Dept. of Education Distributed by Education Publications Center, U.S. Dept. of Education. xii, 124 p.

205. Sacerdote, B., *Peer effects with random assignment: Results for Dartmouth roommates*. Quarterly Journal of Economics, 2000. 116: p. 681. Available from: https://www.nber.org/papers/w7469.pdf.

206. Burdick-Will, J., *School Violent Crime and Academic Achievement in Chicago.* . J. Sociol Educ., 2013. **86**(4). Available from: https://www.ncbi.nlm.nih.gov/pmc/articles/PMC3831577/.

207. McCoy DC, Roy AL, and S. GM., *Neighborhood crime and school climate as predictors of elementary school academic quality: a cross-lagged panel analysis*. Am J Community Psychol., 2013. **52**(1-2): p. 128-40. Available from: https://www.ncbi.nlm.nih.gov/pubmed/23764745.

208. Lacoe, J., *Unequally Safe: The Race Gap in School Safety*. Youth Violence and Juvenile Justice, 2015. **13**(2): p. 143-168.

209. Division of Adolescent and School Health. *National Center for HIV/AIDS, V.H., STD, and TB Prevention. Centers for Disease Control and Prevention, YOUTH RISK BEHAVIOR SURVEY. DATA SUMMARY & TRENDS REPORT 2007–2017*. Journal.; Available from: https://www.cdc.gov/healthyyouth/data/yrbs/pdf/trendsreport.pdf.

210. Sharkey, P., et al., *High Stakes in the Classroom, High Stakes on the Street: The Effects of Community Violence on students' Standardized Test Performance*. Sociological Science 2014. 1: p. 199-220. Available from: https://www.sociologicalscience.com/download/volume%201/may(3)/high-stakes-in-the-classroom-high-stakes-on-the-street.pdf.

211. U.S. Department of Education, O.f.C.R., *Securing Equal Educational Opportunity: Report to the President and Secretary of Education Under Section 203(b)(1) of the Department of Education Organization Act, FY 2016. Journal, 2016*. Available from: https://www2.ed.gov/about/reports/annual/ocr/report-to-president-and-secretary-of-education-2016.pdf.

212. Margolin, J., et al., *What Factors Predict the Success of Hispanic Students in Postsecondary STEM Majors?, in Annual Meeting of the American Educational Research Association 2018, AERA online paper repository: New York City, NY*. Available from: http://www.aera.net/Publications/Online-Paper-Repository/AERA-Online-Paper-Repository.

213. Johnson, R. *In Search of Integration: Beyond Black & White*. 2014. Available from: https://furmancenter.org/research/iri/essay/in-search-of-integration-beyond-black-white.

214. Hughes, J.N., et al., *Effect of Early Grade Retention on School Completion: A Prospective Study*. J Educ Psychol, 2018. **110**(7): p. 974-991. Available from: https://www.ncbi.nlm.nih.gov/pubmed/30778263.

215. Balfanz, R. and N. Legters, *Locating the dropout crisis. Which High Schools produce the nation's dropouts? Where are they located? who attends them?* Journal, 2004. Available from: https://files.eric.ed.gov/fulltext/ED484525.pdf.

216. Rendon, L.I., *Validating culturally diverse students: Toward a new model of learning and student development*. Innovative Higher Education, 1994. **19**(1):

p. 33-51. Available from: https://doi.org/10.1007/BF01191156   https://www.csuchico.edu/ourdemocracy/_assets/documents/pedagogy/rendon,-l.-1994---validation-theory.pdf.

217. Broton, K.M., *Rethinking the Cooling Out Hypothesis for the 21st Century: The Impact of Financial Aid on Students' Educational Goals*. Community College Review, 2019. **47**(1): p. 79-104. Available from: https://doi.org/10.1177/0091552118820449.

218. Schmit, S. and C. Walker, *Disparate Access/ Head Start and CCDBG data by race and ethnicity*. Journal, 2016. Available from: https://www.clasp.org/sites/default/files/public/resources-and-publications/publication-1/Disparate-Access.pdf.

219. Silver, J.K., et al., *Physician Workforce Disparities and Patient Care: A Narrative Review. Health Equity,* 2019. **3**(1): p. 360-377. Available from: https://www.ncbi.nlm.nih.gov/pubmed/31312783.

220. Carnethon, M.R., et al., *Association of cardiovascular risk factors between Hispanic/Latino parents and youth: the Hispanic Community Health Study/Study of Latino Youth*. Ann Epidemiol, 2017. **27**(4): p. 260-268 e2. Available from: https://www.ncbi.nlm.nih.gov/pubmed/28476328.

221. Daviglus, M.L., A. Pirzada, and G.A. Talavera, *Cardiovascular disease risk factors in the Hispanic/Latino population: lessons from the Hispanic Community Health Study/Study of Latinos (HCHS/SOL)*. Prog Cardiovasc Dis, 2014. **57**(3): p. 230-6. Available from: https://www.ncbi.nlm.nih.gov/pubmed/25242694.

222. Daviglus, M.L., et al., *Prevalence of major cardiovascular risk factors and cardiovascular diseases among Hispanic/Latino individuals of diverse backgrounds in the United States*. JAMA, 2012. **308**(17): p. 1775-84. Available from: https://www.ncbi.nlm.nih.gov/pubmed/23117778.

223. Appuhamy, R. and A. Appuhamy. *Determinants of health (video). 2020*; Available from: https://www.youtube.com/watch?v=zSguDQRjZv0&feature=youtu.be.

224. 224. Prevention., C.f.D.C.a., *Measuring Healthy Days.* . Journal, 2000. Available from: https://www.cdc.gov/hrqol/pdfs/mhd.pdf.

225. Katiria Perez, G. and D. Cruess, *The impact of familism on physical and mental health among Hispanics in the United States.* Health Psychol Rev, 2014. **8**(1): p. 95-127. Available from: https://www.ncbi.nlm.nih.gov/pubmed/25053010.

226. Handtke, O., B. Schilgen, and M. Mosko, *Culturally competent healthcare - A scoping review of strategies implemented in healthcare organizations and a model of culturally competent healthcare provision.* PLoS One, 2019. **14**(7): p. e0219971. Available from: https://www.ncbi.nlm.nih.gov/pubmed/31361783.

227. Shiels, M.S., et al., *Premature mortality from all causes and drug poisonings in the USA according to socioeconomic status and rurality: an analysis of death certificate data by county from 2000-15.* Lancet Public Health, 2019. **4**(2): p. e97-e106. Available from: https://www.ncbi.nlm.nih.gov/pubmed/30655229.

228. Quandt, S.A., et al., *Cholinesterase depression and its association with pesticide exposure across the agricultural season among Latino farmworkers in North Carolina.* Environ Health Perspect, 2010. **118**(5): p. 635-9. Available from: https://www.ncbi.nlm.nih.gov/pubmed/20085857.

229. McCurdy, S.A., et al., *Region of birth, sex, and agricultural work of immigrant Latino farm workers: the MICASA study.* J Agric Saf Health, 2014. **20**(2): p. 79-90. Available from: https://www.ncbi.nlm.nih.gov/pubmed/24897916.

230. Stoecklin-Marois, M., et al., *Heat-related illness knowledge and practices among California hired farm workers in The MICASA Study.* Ind Health, 2013. **51**(1): p. 47-55. Available from: https://www.ncbi.nlm.nih.gov/pubmed/23411756.

231. Xiao, H., et al., *Agricultural work and chronic musculoskeletal pain among Latino farm workers: the MICASA study.* Am J Ind Med, 2013. **56**(2): p. 216-25. Available from: https://www.ncbi.nlm.nih.gov/pubmed/23023585.

232. Goldman, N., *Will the Latino Mortality Advantage Endure? Res Aging,* 2016. **38**(3): p. 263-82. Available from: https://www.ncbi.nlm.nih.gov/pubmed/26966251.

233. Abraido-Lanza, A.F., M.T. Chao, and K.R. Florez, *Do healthy behaviors decline with greater acculturation? Implications for the Latino mortality paradox.* Soc Sci Med, 2005. **61**(6): p. 1243-55. Available from: https://www.ncbi.nlm.nih.gov/pubmed/15970234.

234. Kershaw, K.N., et al., *Relationships of nativity and length of residence in the U.S. with favorable cardiovascular health among Hispanics/Latinos: The Hispanic Community Health Study/Study of Latinos (HCHS/SOL).* Prev Med, 2016. 89: p. 84-89. Available from: https://www.ncbi.nlm.nih.gov/pubmed/27196144.

235. Boen, C.E. and R.A. Hummer, *Longer-but Harder-Lives?: The Hispanic Health Paradox and the Social Determinants of Racial, Ethnic, and Immigrant-Native Health Disparities from Midlife through Late Life.* J Health Soc Behav, 2019. **60**(4): p. 434-452. Available from: https://www.ncbi.nlm.nih.gov/pubmed/31771347.

236. Flores, M.E., et al., *The "Latina epidemiologic paradox": contrasting patterns of adverse birth outcomes in U.S.-born and foreign-born Latinas.* Womens Health Issues, 2012. **22**(5): p. e501-7. Available from: https://www.ncbi.nlm.nih.gov/pubmed/22944904.

237. Sanchez-Vaznaugh, E.V., et al., *Latina Birth Outcomes in California: Not so Paradoxical.* Matern Child Health J, 2016. **20**(9): p. 1849-60. Available from: https://www.ncbi.nlm.nih.gov/pubmed/27023385.

238. Sparks, P.J., *Do biological, sociodemographic, and behavioral characteristics explain racial/ethnic disparities in preterm births?* Soc Sci Med, 2009. **68**(9): p. 1667-75. Available from: https://www.ncbi.nlm.nih.gov/pubmed/19285373.

239. Herd, D., et al., *Community Level Correlates of Low Birthweight Among African American, Hispanic and White Women in California.* Matern Child Health J, 2015. **19**(10): p. 2251-60. Available from: https://www.ncbi.nlm.nih.gov/pubmed/25998311.

240. Sims, M., T.L. Sims, and M.A. Bruce, *Race, ethnicity, concentrated poverty, and low birth weight disparities.* J Natl Black Nurses Assoc, 2008. **19**(1): p. 12-8. Available from: https://www.ncbi.nlm.nih.gov/pubmed/18807774.

241. Rice, W.S., et al., *Disparities in Infant Mortality by Race Among Hispanic and Non-Hispanic Infants.* Matern Child Health J, 2017. **21**(7): p. 1581-1588. Available from: https://www.ncbi.nlm.nih.gov/pubmed/28197819.

242. Cohen, R., M. Martinez, and E. Zammitti, *Health insurance coverage: Early release of estimates from the National Health Interview Survey.* Journal, 2018. Available from: https://www.cdc.gov/nchs/data/nhis/earlyrelease/Insur201808.pdf.

243. Heron, M., *Deaths: Leading Causes for 2017. Journal, 2019.* 686. Available from: https://www.cdc.gov/nchs/data/nvsr/nvsr68/nvsr68_06-508.pdf.

244. Hales, C.M., et al., *Prevalence of Obesity Among Adults and Youth: United States, 2015-2016*. NCHS Data Brief, 2017(288): p. 1-8. Available from: https://www.ncbi.nlm.nih.gov/pubmed/29155689.

245. Ogden, C.L., et al., *Prevalence of Obesity Among Adults, by Household Income and Education - United States, 2011-2014*. MMWR Morb Mortal Wkly Rep, 2017. **66**(50): p. 1369-1373. Available from: https://www.ncbi.nlm.nih.gov/pubmed/29267260.

246. Hanis, C.L., et al., *Diabetes Among Mexican Americans in Starr County, Texas. American Journal of Epidemiology, 1983.* **118**(5): p. 659-672. Available from: https://doi.org/10.1093/oxfordjournals.aje.a113677.

247. Stern, M.P., et al., *Does obesity explain excess prevalence of diabetes among Mexican Americans? Results of the San Antonio heart study. 1983.* **24**(4): p. 272-277. Available from: https://doi.org/10.1007/BF00282712.

248. American Cancer Society, *Cancer facts & Figures for Hispanics/Latinos 2018-2020*. Journal, 2018. Available from: https://www.cancer.org/content/dam/cancer-org/research/cancer-facts-and-statistics/cancer-facts-and-figures-for-hispanics-and-latinos/cancer-facts-and-figures-for-hispanics-and-latinos-2018-2020.pdf.

249. Marquez, I., N. Calman, and C. Crump, *A Framework for Addressing Diabetes-Related Disparities in US Latino Populations*. J Community Health,

2019. **44**(2): p. 412-422. Available from: https://www.ncbi.nlm.nih.gov/pubmed/30264184.

250. Wray, C.J., et al., *The effect of age on race-related breast cancer survival disparities.* Ann Surg Oncol, 2013. **20**(8): p. 2541-7. Available from: https://www.ncbi.nlm.nih.gov/pubmed/23435633.

251. Cragun, D., et al., *Racial disparities in BRCA testing and cancer risk management across a population-based sample of young breast cancer survivors.* Cancer, 2017. 123(13): p. 2497-2505.

252. Lara-Medina F, et al., *Triple-negative breast cancer in Hispanic patients: high prevalence, poor prognosis, and association with menopausal status, body mass index, and parity.* Cancer, 2011. **117**(16): p. 3658-3669. Available from: https://onlinelibrary.wiley.com/doi/full/10.1002/cncr.25961.

253. Maly, R., et al., *Racial/ethnic group differences in treatment decision-making and treatment received among older breast carcinoma patients.* . Cancer, 2006. **106**(4): p. 957-965. Available from: https://acsjournals.onlinelibrary.wiley.com/doi/full/10.1002/cncr.21680.

254. Olshefsky, A.M., et al., *Promoting HIV risk awareness and testing in Latinos living on the U.S.-Mexico border: the Tu No Me Conoces social marketing campaign.* AIDS Educ Prev, 2007. **19**(5): p. 422-35. Available from: https://www.ncbi.nlm.nih.gov/pubmed/17967112.

255. Mathews TJ, H.B., *Total fertility rates by state and race and Hispanic origin: United States, 2017.* . National Vital Statistics Reports. National Center for Health Statistics, 2018. **68**(1).

256. Tavernise, S., *Why Birthrates Among Hispanic Americans Have Plummeted.* The New York Times, 2019(March 7, 2019). Available from: https://www.nytimes.com/2019/03/07/us/us-birthrate-hispanics-latinos.html.

257. Alvira-Hammond, M., *Hispanic women are helping drive the recent decline in the U.S. fertility rate.* National Research Center on Hispanic children & families, 2019. Available from: http://www.hispanicresearchcenter.org/wp-content/uploads/2019/03/Hispanic-fertility-trends-1989-2017.pdf.

258. Daniels K, A.J., *Current contraceptive status among women aged 15–49: United States*, 2015–2017. . NCHS Data Brief, no 327, 2018.

259. Alegria, M., et al., *Prevalence of psychiatric disorders across Latino subgroups in the United States*. Am J Public Health, 2007. **97**(1): p. 68-75. Available from: https://www.ncbi.nlm.nih.gov/pubmed/17138910.

260. Alvarez, K., et al., *Race/ethnicity, nativity, and lifetime risk of mental disorders in US adults*. Soc Psychiatry Psychiatr Epidemiol, 2019. **54**(5): p. 553-565. Available from: https://www.ncbi.nlm.nih.gov/pubmed/30547212.

261. Breslau, J., et al., *Specifying race-ethnic differences in risk for psychiatric disorder in a USA national sample*. Psychol Med, 2006. **36**(1): p. 57-68. Available from: https://www.ncbi.nlm.nih.gov/pubmed/16202191.

262. Heeringa, S.G., et al., *Sample designs and sampling methods for the Collaborative Psychiatric Epidemiology Studies (CPES)*. Int J Methods Psychiatr Res, 2004. **13**(4): p. 221-40. Available from: https://www.ncbi.nlm.nih.gov/pubmed/15719530.

263. Breslau, J., et al., *Lifetime risk and persistence of psychiatric disorders across ethnic groups in the United States*. Psychol Med, 2005. **35**(3): p. 317-27. Available from: https://www.ncbi.nlm.nih.gov/pubmed/15841868.

264. McGuire, T.G. and J. Miranda, *New evidence regarding racial and ethnic disparities in mental health: policy implications*. Health Aff (Millwood), 2008. **27**(2): p. 393-403. Available from: https://www.ncbi.nlm.nih.gov/pubmed/18332495.

265. Iwelunmor, J., V. Newsome, and C.O. Airhihenbuwa, *Framing the impact of culture on health: a systematic review of the PEN-3 cultural model and its application in public health research and interventions*. Ethn Health, 2014. **19**(1): p. 20-46. Available from: https://www.ncbi.nlm.nih.gov/pubmed/24266638.

266. Gurung, R.A.R., *Multicultural approaches to health and wellness in America*. 2014, Santa Barbara, California: Praeger. 2 volumes.

267. Norris, W.M., et al., *Treatment preferences for resuscitation and critical care*

among homeless persons. Chest, 2005. **127**(6): p. 2180-7. Available from: https://www.ncbi.nlm.nih.gov/pubmed/15947335.

268. Partida, Y., *Language barriers and the patient encounter. Virtual Mentor, 2007.* **9**(8): p. 566. Available from: https://www.ncbi.nlm.nih.gov/pubmed/23218152 https://journalofethics.ama-assn.org/sites/journalofethics.ama-assn.org/files/2018-06/msoc1-0708.pdf.

269. Lubrano di Ciccone, B., et al., *Interviewing patients using interpreters in an oncology setting: initial evaluation of a communication skills module.* Ann Oncol, 2010. **21**(1): p. 27-32. Available from: https://www.ncbi.nlm.nih.gov/pubmed/19622593.

270. Kutner M, et al., *The Health Literacy of America's Adults: Results From the 2003 National Assessment of Adult Literacy (NCES 2006–483).* Journal, 2006. Available from: https://nces.ed.gov/pubs2006/2006483.pdf.

271. Becerra, B.J., D. Arias, and M.B. Becerra, *Low Health Literacy among Immigrant Hispanics. J Racial Ethn Health Disparities, 2017.* **4**(3): p. 480-483. Available from: https://www.ncbi.nlm.nih.gov/pubmed/27324821.

272. Elder, J.P., et al., *Health communication in the Latino community: issues and approaches. Annu Rev Public Health, 2009.* 30: p. 227-51. Available from: https://www.ncbi.nlm.nih.gov/pubmed/19296776.

273. Arcury, T.A., et al., *Treating skin disease: self-management behaviors of Latino farmworkers.* J Agromedicine, 2006. **11**(2): p. 27-35. Available from: https://www.ncbi.nlm.nih.gov/pubmed/17135140.

274. U.S. Department of Health and Human Services, *National Action Plan to Improve Health Literacy.* . Journal, 2010. Available from: https://health.gov/our-work/health-literacy/national-action-plan-improve-health-literacy.

275. David, R.A. and M. Rhee, *The impact of language as a barrier to effective health care in an underserved urban Hispanic community.* Mt Sinai J Med, 1998. **65**(5-6): p. 393-7. Available from: https://www.ncbi.nlm.nih.gov/pubmed/9844369.

276. Fletcher, S.W., et al., *Patients' understanding of prescribed drugs. J Community Health, 1979.* **4**(3): p. 183-9. Available from: https://www.ncbi.nlm.nih.gov/pubmed/457923.

277. Hanchak, N.A., et al., *Patient misunderstanding of dosing instructions.* J Gen Intern Med, 1996. **11**(6): p. 325-8. Available from: https://www.ncbi.nlm.nih.gov/pubmed/8803737.

278. Karliner, L.S., et al., *Language barriers and understanding of hospital discharge instructions.* Med Care, 2012. **50**(4): p. 283-9. Available from: https://www.ncbi.nlm.nih.gov/pubmed/22411441.

279. Carrasquillo, O., et al., *Impact of language barriers on patient satisfaction in an emergency department.* J Gen Intern Med, 1999. **14**(2): p. 82-7. Available from: https://www.ncbi.nlm.nih.gov/pubmed/10051778.

280. Manson, A., *Language concordance as a determinant of patient compliance and emergency room use in patients with asthma.* Med Care, 1988. **26**(12): p. 1119-28. Available from: https://www.ncbi.nlm.nih.gov/pubmed/3199910.

281. Woloshin, S., et al., *Language Barriers in Medicine in the United States.* JAMA, 1995. **273**(9): p. 724-728. Available from: https://doi.org/10.1001/jama.1995.03520330054037.

282. Perez-Stable, E.J., A. Napoles-Springer, and J.M. Miramontes, *The effects of ethnicity and language on medical outcomes of patients with hypertension or diabetes.* Med Care, 1997. **35**(12): p. 1212-9. Available from: https://www.ncbi.nlm.nih.gov/pubmed/9413309.

283. Cooper, L.A., et al., *Patient-Centered Communication, Ratings of Care, and Concordance of Patient and Physician Race.* Annals of Internal Medicine, 2003. **139**(11): p. 907-915. Available from: https://doi.org/10.7326/0003-4819-139-11-200312020-00009.

284. Guntzviller, L.M., J.D. Jensen, and L.M. Carreno, *Latino children's ability to interpret in health settings: A parent–child dyadic perspective on child health literacy.* Communication Monographs, 2017. **84**(2): p. 143-163. Available from: https://doi.org/10.1080/03637751.2016.1214871.

285. Aguado Loi, C.X., et al., *Application of mixed-methods design in community-engaged research: Lessons learned from an evidence-based intervention for Latinos with chronic illness and minor depression.* Eval Program Plann, 2017. 63: p. 29-38. Available from: https://www.ncbi.nlm.nih.gov/pubmed/28343021.

286. Rivera, Y.M., et al., *When a Common Language Is Not Enough: Transcreating Cancer 101 for Communities in Puerto Rico.* J Cancer Educ, 2016. **31**(4): p. 776-783. Available from: https://www.ncbi.nlm.nih.gov/pubmed/26365291.

287. Alden, D.L., et al., *The effects of culturally targeted patient decision aids on medical consultation preparation for Hispanic women in the U.S.: Results from four randomized experiments.* Soc Sci Med, 2018. 212: p. 17-25. Available from: https://www.ncbi.nlm.nih.gov/pubmed/29990671.

288. Martinez Tyson, D., et al., *Cultural adaptation of a supportive care needs measure for Hispanic men cancer survivors.* J Psychosoc Oncol, 2018. **36**(1): p. 113-131. Available from: https://www.ncbi.nlm.nih.gov/pubmed/28857692.

289. Saha, S., et al., *Do patients choose physicians of their own race? Health Aff (Millwood),* 2000. **19**(4): p. 76-83. Available from: https://www.ncbi.nlm.nih.gov/pubmed/10916962.

290. LaVeist, T.A. and A. Nuru-Jeter, *Is Doctor-Patient Race Concordance Associated with Greater Satisfaction with Care? Journal of Health and Social Behavior,* 2002. **43**(3): p. 296-306. Available from: www.jstor.org/stable/3090205.

291. Lopez, S., A. Lopez, and K. Fong, *Mexican Americans' initial preferences for counselors: The role of ethnic factors.* Journal of Counseling Psychology 1991. **38**(4): p. 487–496.

292. Moy, E. and B.A. Bartman, *Physician Race and Care of Minority and Medically Indigent Patients.* JAMA, 1995. **273**(19): p. 1515-1520. Available from: https://doi.org/10.1001/jama.1995.03520430051038.

293. Walker, K.O., G. Moreno, and K. Grumbach, *The association among specialty, race, ethnicity, and practice location among California physicians in diverse specialties.* J Natl Med Assoc, 2012. **104**(1-2): p. 46-52. Available from: https://www.ncbi.nlm.nih.gov/pubmed/22708247.

294. Saha, S., et al., *Patient-physician racial concordance and the perceived quality and use of health care.* Arch Intern Med, 1999. **159**(9): p. 997-1004. Available from: https://www.ncbi.nlm.nih.gov/pubmed/10326942.

295. Marrast, L.M., et al., *Minority physicians' role in the care of underserved patients: diversifying the physician workforce may be key in addressing health disparities.* JAMA Intern Med, 2014. **174**(2): p. 289-91. Available from: https://www.ncbi.nlm.nih.gov/pubmed/24378807.

296. The University of Chicago. *National Survey of Early Care and Education.* Available from: https://www.norc.org/Research/Projects/Pages/national-survey-of-early-care-and-education.aspx.

297. Todd, K.H., et al., *Ethnicity and analgesic practice.* Ann Emerg Med, 2000. **35**(1): p. 11-6. Available from: https://www.ncbi.nlm.nih.gov/pubmed/10613935.

298. Heins, A., et al., *Physician race/ethnicity predicts successful emergency department analgesia.* J Pain, 2010. **11**(7): p. 692-7. Available from: https://www.ncbi.nlm.nih.gov/pubmed/20382572.

299. Todd, K.H., N. Samaroo, and J.R. Hoffman, *Ethnicity as a risk factor for inadequate emergency department analgesia.* JAMA, 1993. **269**(12): p. 1537-9. Available from: https://www.ncbi.nlm.nih.gov/pubmed/8445817.

300. Udyavar, N.R., et al., *Do outcomes in emergency general surgery vary for minority patients based on surgeons' racial/ethnic case mix?* Am J Surg, 2019. **218**(1): p. 42-46. Available from: https://www.ncbi.nlm.nih.gov/pubmed/30711193.

301. Adelekun, A.A., et al., *Recognizing Racism in Medicine: A Student-Organized and Community-Engaged Health Professional Conference.* Health Equity, 2019. **3**(1): p. 395-402. Available from: https://www.ncbi.nlm.nih.gov/pubmed/31406953.

302. Beach, M.C., et al., *Cultural competence: a systematic review of health care provider educational interventions.* Med Care, 2005. **43**(4): p. 356-73. Available from: https://www.ncbi.nlm.nih.gov/pubmed/15778639.

303. Loudon, R.F., et al., *Educating medical students for work in culturally diverse societies*. JAMA, 1999. **282**(9): p. 875-80. Available from: https://www.ncbi.nlm.nih.gov/pubmed/10478695.

304. Truong, M., Y. Paradies, and N. Priest, *Interventions to improve cultural competency in healthcare: a systematic review of reviews*. BMC Health Serv Res, 2014. 14: p. 99. Available from: https://www.ncbi.nlm.nih.gov/pubmed/24589335.

305. American Hospital Association, *Does your hospital reflect the community it serves? A Diversity and Cultural Proficiency Assessment Tool for Leaders Journal, 2004*. Available from: https://www.aana.com/docs/default-source/about-us-aana.com-web-documents-(all)/aha-strategies-for-leadership_a-diversity-and-cultural-proficiency-assessmen-_.pdf?sfvrsn=bc3a42b1_10.

306. Lie, D.A., et al., *Does cultural competency training of health professionals improve patient outcomes? A systematic review and proposed algorithm for future research*. J Gen Intern Med, 2011. **26**(3): p. 317-25. Available from: https://www.ncbi.nlm.nih.gov/pubmed/20953728.

307. Rudman, L.A., R.D. Ashmore, and M.L. Gary, *"Unlearning" automatic biases: The malleability of implicit prejudice and stereotypes*. Journal of Personality and Social Psychology, 2001. **81**(5): p. 856-868. Available from: https://psycnet.apa.org/record/2001-05123-009.

308. McElmurry, B.J., et al., *Implementation, outcomes, and lessons learned from a collaborative primary health care program to improve diabetes care among urban Latino populations*. Health Promot Pract, 2009. **10**(2): p. 293-302. Available from: https://www.ncbi.nlm.nih.gov/pubmed/18344318.

309. Shepherd, S.M., *Cultural awareness workshops: limitations and practical consequences*. BMC Med Educ, 2019. **19**(1): p. 14. Available from: https://www.ncbi.nlm.nih.gov/pubmed/30621665.

310. Noon, M., *Pointless Diversity Training: Unconscious Bias, New Racism and Agency*. 2018. **32**(1): p. 198-209. Available from: https://journals.sagepub.com/doi/abs/10.1177/0950017017719841.

311. Fernandez-Gutierrez, M., et al., *Health literacy interventions for immigrant populations: a systematic review*. Int Nurs Rev, 2018. **65**(1): p. 54-64. Available from: https://www.ncbi.nlm.nih.gov/pubmed/28449363.

312. Chaufan, C., et al., *Identifying Spanish Language Competent Physicians: The Diabetes Study of Northern California (DISTANCE)*. Ethn Dis, 2016. **26**(4): p. 537-544. Available from: https://www.ncbi.nlm.nih.gov/pubmed/27773981.

313. Betancourt, J., et al., *Improving Patient Safety Systems for Patients With Limited English Proficiency*. A Guide for Hospitals. Journal, 2012. Available from: https://www.ahrq.gov/sites/default/files/publications/files/lepguide.pdf.

314. Karliner, L.S., *Protocols can lead to equitable emergency cardiac care for patients with language barriers, but quality communication remains important for access, outcomes and prevention*. Eur Heart J Qual Care Clin Outcomes, 2020. Available from: https://www.ncbi.nlm.nih.gov/pubmed/31999313.

315. Brown, S., et al., *Culturally competent diabetes self-management education for Mexican Americans: the Starr County border health initiative*. Diabetes Care, 2002. **25**(2): p. 259-268. Available from: https://care.diabetesjournals.org/content/25/2/259.long.

316. Rickheim, P., et al., *Assessment of Group Versus Individual Diabetes Education. A Randomized Study*. Diabetes Care, 2002. 25: p. 269-274. Available from: https://care.diabetesjournals.org/content/diacare/25/2/269.full.pdf.

317. Foreyt, J., A. Ramirez, and J. Hays, *Cuidando El Corazon - A weight-reduction intervention for Mexican Americans*. The American journal of clinical nutrition, 1991. 53: p. 1639S-1641S.

318. Olson, R., F. Sabogal, and A. Perez, *Viva La Vida: Helping Latino Medicare Beneficiaries With Diabetes Live Their Lives to the Fullest*. American Journal of Public Health, 2008. 98: p. 205-208. Available from: https://ajph.aphapublications.org/doi/pdf/10.2105/AJPH.2006.106062.

319. Elder, J.P., et al., *Long-term effects of a communication intervention for Spanish-dominant Latinas*. Am J Prev Med, 2006. **31**(2): p. 159-66. Available from: https://www.ncbi.nlm.nih.gov/pubmed/16829333.

320. Elder, J.P., et al., *Interpersonal and print nutrition communication for a Spanish-dominant Latino population: Secretos de la Buena Vida*. Health Psychol, 2005. **24**(1): p. 49-57. Available from: https://www.ncbi.nlm.nih.gov/pubmed/15631562.

321. Baquero, B., et al., *Secretos de la Buena Vida: processes of dietary change via a tailored nutrition communication intervention for Latinas*. Health Educ Res, 2009. **24**(5): p. 855-66. Available from: https://www.ncbi.nlm.nih.gov/pubmed/19339374.

322. Cameron, L.D., et al., *Cultural and Linguistic Adaptation of a Healthy Diet Text Message Intervention for Hispanic Adults Living in the United States*. J Health Commun, 2017. **22**(3): p. 262-273. Available from: https://www.ncbi.nlm.nih.gov/pubmed/28248628.

323. Thompson, B., et al., *Celebremos la salud! a community randomized trial of cancer prevention (United States)*. Cancer Causes Control, 2006. **17**(5): p. 733-746.

324. Tejeda, S., et al., *Celebremos la Salud: a community-based intervention for Hispanic and non-Hispanic white women living in a rural area. J Community Health, 2009*. **34**(1): p. 47-55. Available from: https://www.ncbi.nlm.nih.gov/pubmed/18821000.

325. Scheel, J.R., et al., *Latinas' Mammography Intention Following a Home-Based Promotores-Led Intervention*. J Community Health, 2015. **40**(6): p. 1185-92. Available from: https://www.ncbi.nlm.nih.gov/pubmed/26063674.

326. Livaudais, J.C., et al., *Educating Hispanic women about breast cancer prevention: evaluation of a home-based promotora-led intervention. J Womens Health (Larchmt), 2010*. **19**(11): p. 2049-56. Available from: https://www.ncbi.nlm.nih.gov/pubmed/20849288.

327. Molina, Y., et al., *Breast cancer interventions serving US-based Latinas: current approaches and directions*. Womens Health (Lond), 2013. 9(4): p. 335-48; quiz 349-50. Available from: https://www.ncbi.nlm.nih.gov/pubmed/23826775.

328. Cupertino, A.P., et al., *Empowering Promotores de Salud to engage in Community-Based Participatory Research*. J Immigr Refug Stud, 2013. **11**(1): p. 24-43. Available from: https://www.ncbi.nlm.nih.gov/pubmed/25705141.

329. Larkey, L., *Las mujeres saludables: reaching Latinas for breast, cervical and colorectal cancer prevention and screening*. J Community Health, 2006. **31**(1): p. 69-77. Available from: https://www.ncbi.nlm.nih.gov/pubmed/16482767.

330. Welsh, A.L., et al., *The effect of two church-based interventions on breast cancer screening rates among Medicaid-insured Latinas*. Prev Chronic Dis, 2005. **2**(4): p. A07. Available from: https://www.ncbi.nlm.nih.gov/pubmed/16164811.

331. Sauaia, A., et al., *Church-based breast cancer screening education: impact of two approaches on Latinas enrolled in public and private health insurance plans*. Prev Chronic Dis, 2007. **4**(4): p. A99. Available from: https://www.ncbi.nlm.nih.gov/pubmed/17875274.

332. Barnack-Tavlaris, J., et al., *Abstract A20: Increasing pap testing with a community-based educational intervention in the Latina population*. Cancer Epidemiol Biomarkers Prev, 2010. 19: p. A20.

333. Navarro, A., et al., *Por La Vida model intervention enhances use of cancer screening tests among Latinas*. American Journal of Preventive Medicine, 1998. **15**(1). Available from: https://www.ajpmonline.org/article/S0749-3797(98)00023-3/abstract.

334. Ramirez, A.G. and A.L. McAlister, *Mass media campaign--A Su Salud*. Prev Med, 1988. **17**(5): p. 608-21. Available from: https://www.ncbi.nlm.nih.gov/pubmed/3237659.

335. Wetter, D.W., et al., *Reaching and treating Spanish-speaking smokers through the National Cancer Institute's Cancer Information Service. A randomized controlled trial*. Cancer, 2007. **109**(2 Suppl): p. 406-13. Available from: https://www.ncbi.nlm.nih.gov/pubmed/17149758.

336. Squiers, L., et al., *Cancer patients' information needs across the cancer care continuum: evidence from the cancer information service*. J Health Commun,

2005. 10 Suppl 1: p. 15-34. Available from: https://www.ncbi.nlm.nih.gov/pubmed/16377598.

337. Elder, J.P., et al., *Tobacco and alcohol use-prevention program for Hispanic migrant adolescents*. Am J Prev Med, 2002. **23**(4): p. 269-75. Available from: https://www.ncbi.nlm.nih.gov/pubmed/12406481.

338. Yancey, A.K., et al., *Increased cancer screening behavior in women of color by culturally sensitive video exposure*. Prev Med, 1995. **24**(2): p. 142-8. Available from: https://www.ncbi.nlm.nih.gov/pubmed/7597016.

339. Yancey, A.K. and L. Walden, *Stimulating cancer screening among Latinas and African-American women: A community case study*. Journal of Cancer Education, 1994. **9**(1): p. 46-52. Available from: https://www.tandfonline.com/doi/abs/10.1080/08858199409528265.

340. Wilkin, H.A., et al., *Does entertainment-education work with Latinos in the United States? Identification and the effects of a telenovela breast cancer storyline*. J Health Commun, 2007. **12**(5): p. 455-69. Available from: https://www.ncbi.nlm.nih.gov/pubmed/17710596.

341. Caicedo, L., K. BrintzenhofeSzoc, and J. Zabora, *Abstract B18: Impact of Nueva Vida's model on self-efficacy in Latinas with breast cancer, in AACR International Conference on the Science of Cancer Health Disparities*. 2010, Behavioral and Social Science: Miami, FL. Available from: https://cebp.aacrjournals.org/content/19/10_Supplement/B18.

342. Patel, T.A., et al., *Breast cancer in Latinas: gene expression, differential response to treatments, and differential toxicities in Latinas compared with other population groups*. Oncologist, 2010. **15**(5): p. 466-75. Available from: https://www.ncbi.nlm.nih.gov/pubmed/20427382.

343. Lopez, M. *Three-Fourths of Hispanics Say Their Community Needs a Leader. Most Latinos Cannot Name One*. 2013. Available from: https://www.pewresearch.org/hispanic/2013/10/22/three-fourths-of-hispanics-say-their-community-needs-a-leader/.

344. Gordon, E.J., et al., *Hispanic/Latino Disparities in Living Donor Kidney Transplantation: Role of a Culturally Competent Transplant Program.* Transplant Direct, 2015. **1**(8): p. e29. Available from: https://www.ncbi.nlm.nih.gov/pubmed/27500229.

345. Gordon, E.J., et al., *Culturally competent transplant program improves Hispanics' knowledge and attitudes about live kidney donation and transplant.* Prog Transplant, 2014. **24**(1): p. 56-68. Available from: https://www.ncbi.nlm.nih.gov/pubmed/24598567.

346. Tam, I., et al., *Spanish Interpreter Services for the Hospitalized Pediatric Patient: Provider and Interpreter Perceptions.* Acad Pediatr, 2020. **20**(2): p. 216-224. Available from: https://www.ncbi.nlm.nih.gov/pubmed/31445969.

347. Soares, L., *Post-traditional Learners and the Transformation of Postsecondary Education: A Manifesto for College Leaders.* Journal, 2013. Available from: http://louissoares.com/wp-content/uploads/2013/02/post_traditional_learners.pdf.

348. Bean, J.P. and B.S. Metzner, *A Conceptual Model of Nontraditional Undergraduate Student Attrition.* Review of Educational Research, 1985. **55**(4): p. 485-540. Available from: www.jstor.org/stable/1170245.

349. National Center for Education Statistics. *Nontraditional Undergraduates / Definitions and Data.* Available from: https://nces.ed.gov/pubs/web/97578d.asp.

350. Rubin, R. *Will the Real SMART Goals Please Stand Up? The Industrial-Organizational Psychologist, 2004.* 4. Available from: http://citeseerx.ist.psu.edu/viewdoc/download?doi=10.1.1.523.6999&rep=rep1&type=pdf.

351. Locke, E.A., *Toward a theory of task motivation and incentives. Organizational Behavior and Human Performance,* 1968. **3**(2): p. 157-189. Available from: http://www.sciencedirect.com/science/article/pii/0030507368900044.

352. Drucker, P.F., *The practice of management. 1st Perennial Library ed.* 1986, New York: Perennial Library. xii, 404 p.; Available from: https://www.harpercollins.com/9780060878979/the-practice-of-management/.

www.ingramcontent.com/pod-product-compliance
Lightning Source LLC
Chambersburg PA
CBHW070908030426
42336CB00014BA/2336